PRAISE FOR C

"I very much appreciated ˌ.̣ˌaᵗ you did for your daughter. You exhibited survival behavior and sought to achieve your daughter's potential to heal. You are an example for others to follow when confronted by adversity."

> —**Bernie Siegel, M.D.**, Author, *Love, Medicine and Miracles* and *A Book of Miracles* w/ **Deepak Chopra**

"The empowering story of a mother's courage in embracing holistic therapies when standard treatments offered no answers. I am proud to have helped kindle Denise's interest in natural medicine nearly three decades ago!"

> —**Ronald Hoffman, M.D.**, Author, Founder and Medical Director of the Hoffman Center in New York, Host of *"Health Talk,"* nationally syndicated radio talk show

"Over the course of my career, a few patients stand out above all the others. Courtney, a 12-year-old girl back in 2007, was one of those patients that brought tears to my eyes when we met. She was looking down the barrel of a very dangerous, potentially life threatening disease, Autoimmune Hepatitis, and she was running out of options fast. Traditional medicine didn't have all the answers in her case, and she continued to lose ground over the five year period when she was doing everything that modern medicine had to offer. Sometimes we forget to summon the doctor within to participate in our road to recovery. I have always taught that to have a chance at "curing" any long term, chronic illness, you must address the diet, food intolerances, support the immune system with specific vitamins, minerals, herbs and utilizing natural protocols when appropriate. I was so excited to see Courtney turn the corner after she started to change her approach and take a more natural path, with me as well as using the protocol of the esteemed Dr. Burt Berkson and his ALA treatments. The results speak loud and clear of the importance of being open minded and never quitting.

The mom, Denise, is an angel and every kid going through the hell that Courtney was in should have a mom that was willing to fight that hard. **Her love for Courtney was the catalyst in making their "miracle" a reality."**

—**Douglas Willen, D.C.**, CEO of Willen Wellness in NYC, Author, Quantum Paleo

Denise Gabay Otten's courageous search for treatments for her daughter's very serious illness took her outside the domain of conventional medicine. Her dedication is a shining example of how a mother can use her love and her research skills to save her child's life. Denise followed her heart—and her gut—and a healthy, happy Courtney is the result!

—**Julia Schopick**, Author, *Honest Medicine: Effective, Time-Tested, Inexpensive Treatments for Life-Threatening Diseases*

I met Denise when she worked at CNBC and I was a regularly scheduled guest commentator on commodity markets. At that time, we shared an interest in healthful living and holistic approaches to wellness before it was fashionable. Interestingly, Courtney's story shares a common thread with my own daughter, Rikki, who developed an "incurable" skin infection from a cast on her broken leg. My pursuit of a better answer than amputation led me to a colloidal silver gel that eliminated the disease and left only a reminding scar. Denise' story of a mother's undaunted efforts to confront and overcome a deadly condition is important for everyone. We can never know if and when we might face a similar situation for a loved one or ourselves. Knowing that there are powerful and successful alternatives to conventional approaches can make the difference between life and death or joy or devastation. I encourage everyone to read, learn, and apply the principles outlined in this blow-by-blow account and ultimate success story.

—**Philip Gotthelf**, President of Equidex, Author, *Commodex* and *Currency Trading: How To Access And Trade The World's Biggest Market*

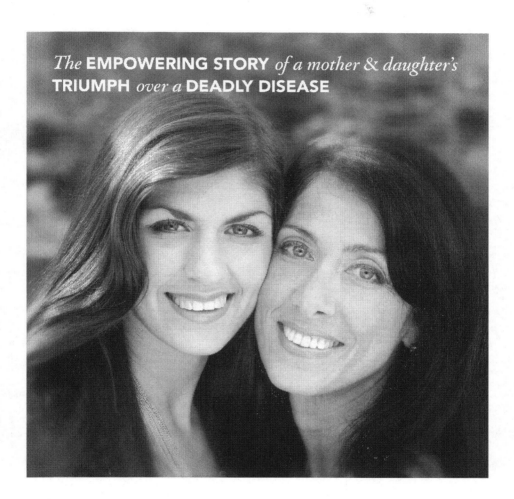

The **EMPOWERING STORY** *of a mother & daughter's* **TRIUMPH** *over a* **DEADLY DISEASE**

Doctors Couldn't Save Her
...So Her Mom Did

Curing Courtney

Denise Gabay Otten

CURING COURTNEY Doctors Couldn't Save Her, So Her Mom Did
by Denise Gabay Otten

Published by Manifesting Life Publishing
www.curingcourtney.com

Author Services by Pedernales Publishing, LLC.
www.pedernalespublishing.com

Editor: Barbara Ardinger, PhD

Cover Design: George Foster, Foster Covers, www.fostercovers.com

Front and Back Photos by: Anthony Grasso Photography,
www.grassophotography.com

Make-up/Hair for Book Cover: Terese Broccoli, www.teresebroccoli.com

All other photos are by Denise Otten except the following:
p. 27 Lifetouch School Portraits
p. 28 Daniel Goscicki
P. 126 Alexandra Wildmoser-Todd

To buy books in quantity for corporate use or for special promotions, go to
www.curingcourtney.com or contact the author at dotten@curingcourtney.com.

Author's note: I have tried to recreate events, locales and conversations from
my memories of them. In order to maintain their anonymity in some instances
I have changed the names of individuals and places, I may have changed some
identifying characteristics and details such as physical properties, occupations
and places of residence.

ISBN 978-0-9886461-1-7

Printed in the United States of America

DEDICATION

To my glorious family—Michael, Adam and Cara.
Without their love and faith in their mother and wife,
my search for Courtney's healing
would not have happened.
And to...
my Beautiful Baby Girl, Courtney Paige,
whose joyous life is a testament to a child's
desire to live large
every day
and to the fact that...
a mother's love can move mountains
and a human spirit believes it will heal!

DISCLAIMER

The health information given in this book is based solely on the personal experience of the author. This book should not be interpreted as medical advice or instruction. The information should not be used for diagnosis or treatment or as a substitute for professional medical care.

Readers are urged to seek the advice of their physicians or health care providers prior to attempting treatment for themselves or other persons.

TABLE OF CONTENTS

Curing Courtney

FOREWORD

How I Learned to Treat Liver Disease
By Burton M. Berkson, M.D., M.S., Ph.D

Thirty-five years ago, when I was an internal medicine resident at a university-affiliated hospital in Cleveland, I was given two patients who had severely poisoned their livers. The chief of medicine told me that the university liver expert said that the patients would die within two weeks because no liver transplants were available. A few weeks earlier, a young girl had died from the same disease, and her father was very ill with the same problem. The chief told me that nothing could be done for these two new patients and I should watch them go through the various stages of liver death and report this information to grand medical rounds in two weeks. He also told me that these patients were my responsibility and would surely die.

I had been a professor of biology with an M.D. and a Ph.D. prior to doing the hospital work to obtain training in internal medicine. A Ph.D. scientist always looks for new information, so I called the

National Institutes of Health (NIH) in Washington, D.C., and asked to talk to the head doctor, F. C. Bartter, M.D. I asked him if he knew of any drug that might stimulate the regeneration of a liver. He told me that he was studying alpha lipoic acid (ALA) as a wonder drug for the reversal of diabetic complications. When a patient was given ALA, he seemed to regenerate his liver and other organs. Dr. Bartter then sent me some ALA. I picked it up at the airport from a commercial pilot and hurried back to the hospital to administer it to my dying patients. I was very excited to see how effective this agent would be. Within two weeks, these patients had regenerated their livers. Both patients are still alive today without any liver problems.

The doctors in D.C. were very interested in my work and sent a team to Cleveland to examine my patients. But the chiefs at the hospital were angry. "How dare you use a drug that was not approved by our pharmacy committee?" they asked. This committee did not meet for another month.

After the FDA appointed me the chief investigator for ALA as a drug, Dr. Bartter and I gave it to seventy-nine people who were dying of acute liver disease. Seventy-five regenerated their livers. I was surprised, however, that there was no interest in ALA in the United States. The hospitals were more interested in transplanting livers rather than in regrowing them. In addition, drug companies were not interested because ALA is natural and cannot easily be patented. The drug also had too many indications. If it was given for liver disease, it would also lower blood sugars and interfere with the sales of insulin and other drugs. Over the years, I started using ALA for hepatitis C, B, autoimmune hepatitis, autoimmune disease, diabetes, and some forms of cancer, all with the same amazing results.

Dr. Bartter and I were invited to be visiting scientists in Germany, where our papers were published.

In this excellent book, Denise Otten describes how her beautiful young daughter, Courtney, developed autoimmune hepatitis, and the doctors at prestigious institutions did not know how to effectively treat her with the standard drugs. Courtney was given prednisone, which blew her up like a balloon, interfered with her normal immunity, caused her bones to become soft, and made her even sicker.

Denise learned about my work with ALA from a woman she met via the Internet and immediately phoned my office in Las Cruces, New Mexico. Courtney was weaned off the prednisone and given ALA and other simple and relatively inexpensive supplements. Today she is a healthy and beautiful teenager who does not want to look back at the damaging therapies she was given by the so-called experts in hepatology.

One wonders why the medical establishment does not accept a new drug when there is so much research to prove that it is efficacious. As Dr. Julian Whitaker wrote in the foreword to one of my books, *The Alpha Lipoic Acid Breakthrough,*

> *"When I was in medical school in the mid-1960's, I was convinced that the medical profession was pure. I was convinced the profession and all those in it were driven by the natural inclination to alleviate suffering and disease. I was convinced that the mere suggestion of patient benefit from therapies not commonly used, such as acupuncture, coenzyme Q10, alpha lipoic acid, chiropractic, or vitamin C, would be quickly examined in an unbiased fashion and would be incorporated if found to be helpful. I was proud of my chosen profession.*

> *Today, thirty years later, the profession embarrasses me. I now realize that the majority of physicians who make up the profession, particularly those in positions of power and authority, have no intention of investigating therapies other than those from pharmaceutical manufacturers. In fact, as macabre as it may seem, many physicians would rather that their patients die than be saved by an unconventional approach. That fact is obvious."*

After practicing medicine for thirty-five years, I believe that Dr. Whitaker's words are correct.

Burton M. Berkson, M.D., M.S., Ph.D.
President, The Integrative Medical Center of New Mexico
Las Cruces, New Mexico

PREFACE

Can We Talk?

By Lynn Doyle, Emmy Award Winning Journalist

As a journalist for more than thirty years, I have covered many heartbreaking stories and been witness to individuals facing devastating loss. But I have also been inspired by the incredible faith people have, their determination to overcome challenges, and their belief that love truly can conquer all. All these elements came together for me almost a decade ago, when my very dear friend, Denise Gabay Otten, revealed to me that her precious daughter Courtney had been diagnosed with a life-threatening illness at the tender age of seven. It was heart-wrenching to watch Denise struggle to accept this diagnosis, and I could find very few words of comfort to offer. What can one say to a mother who is facing the loss of her child? In the end, this mother, my friend, refused to accept the diagnosis and with the same commitment and doggedness that compelled her to success in the business world, she tackled her daughter's illness. In her book, she recounts the horror of facing her child's potential death and, in compelling details, reveals the callousness of those in the medical field. "Accept it," they told her. "Deal with it," others said. "Forget alternatives, they're for quacks," they advised. "You're crazy," some even smirked. But Denise forged on. Her belief in alternative, holistic medicine was genuine. But it was her belief in her own instincts that truly empowered her. And the results were life-saving. *Curing Courtney: Doctors Couldn't Save Her...So Her Mom Did* is an inspiring story of a mother who would not give up on her daughter's life. It's a story of hope for others facing a similar loss too painful for words. And it's a look into the heart and soul of a woman who would not take no for an answer when it came to saving her child's life. This is a woman I am proud to call my friend.

INTRODUCTION

My Daughter Has Autoimmune WHAT? WTF?

Why in the world would you read my story of how I saved my daughter's life from a deadly autoimmune disease, and how we beat the medical odds?

I'm a warrior mother. I'm not a rock star who recovered from breast cancer via chemotherapy treatment or a blonde starlet who was healed of hepatitis C after taking interferon. I'm an ordinary suburban, New Jersey mom (though I'm originally from New York City) who didn't listen to the top New York doctors. I'm a mother who healed my daughter's autoimmune hepatitis using holistic treatments. Now my daughter Courtney is tall, healthy, gorgeous, and athletic. You can see her in the photos in this book.

I'm a "softball and volleyball mom" (but not a soccer mom) who's intensely committed to the health and happiness of my children, just like millions of American women, and my husband is a great father, just like millions of American men. I'm a city girl and he's a country boy and we're living the American dream. We've worked hard and bought our dream house. We're bringing up three beautiful kids. Does this sound just like you, except in a different city? We really are like you...except for one small difference. I healed my baby girl of a life threatening disease, and I did it the natural way. Yes, that's right. I did this after she underwent five years of a failed treatment at one of the top New York pediatric hospitals. She was diagnosed at age seven, and by the time she was twelve years old, the doctors were essentially telling me their standard protocols weren't working and Courtney would need more powerful drugs. I told them NO. Then I did a lot of on-line research and found a scientifically proven, alternative treatment.

I've always been a little pushier than the average gal. I'm a true New Yorker—I try to get what I want and I don't take no for an answer. Though I don't want to be obnoxious about it. Well, this time my relentless persistence paid off. Read on and be amazed at how a mother's tenacity and love healed her daughter's fatal illness.

No, I'm not a physician or a medical practitioner. I'm a financial advisor who manages millions of dollars in my own wealth advisory firm. And I love my kids more than my own life. I know many of you do, too. So when I started this book in 2008, I caught a lot of flak from some of my friends and family. I was put down and belittled by people who said they were my friends. Who, they asked, is going to read a book or listen to an ordinary New Jersey mom who doesn't have a medical degree?

I secretly imagined that millions of people who have open minds and are eager to learn about honest medicine and healthy living will read this book. For years I allowed people to influence me and quash my dreams of telling the world about my personal miracle, and my passion to help other children and adults with autoimmune hepatitis (AIH) and other autoimmune diseases. Because I was getting no support, I put down my dream of writing this book and just quietly tended to my family and clients.

As Courtney grew healthier and more beautiful during the past four years, I started writing again. I wrote a few pages every month, almost like keeping a diary, so I wouldn't forget this devastating time in our life. After my fiftieth birthday, I realized, as many of us do, that I really do have something to offer the world. I'll be darned if one more person tells me I don't have enough initials after my name to write a book and have it published for people to read. If I can open parents' minds and save one child's life, then this book is worth writing and reading. I've also found a reason why my Courtney had to go through this horrible ordeal.

My mother always told me that women can

make a difference in the world. We can do it one woman at a time. Mom brought my sisters and me up in the 1970s during the era of the Equal Rights Amendment (ERA) and instilled in us the belief that with hard work and determination you can achieve anything in life. But what I've discovered was that when others knock you down emotionally and suggest that you don't have the educational level to write a book or contribute to the health of children everywhere, it's hard to speak out and do something against societal norms.

It's especially difficult when you're opposing what the U.S. Food and Drug Administration (FDA) and the American Medical Association (AMA) declare to be established scientific fact. Well, I'm here to tell you—I'm making a difference! And I'm starting it with this book. I know Courtney's story will help you and your family and friends, if not helping you reverse a disease, then by giving you the courage and inner strength to do some research and find your own cures.

I'm not going to boastfully say that I have the alternative answers to every disease. If anyone tells you that, turn around and run away. As fast as possible. No one person knows everything about the human body. But if I have found a holistic treatment that has brought a deadly autoimmune disease into remission for three people—and these people are described in this book—don't you think it's in your best interest to find out how I did it and where I found the scientific research to validate the protocol? Read on and get ready to change your mind set. Or at least, learn a lot.

Since I started doing my own research in 2007, I've found several ways to heal autoimmune diseases. This is the story of just one protocol and one kid who is alive because of what I learned. There are many other doctors and laymen who have nutritional answers to other deadly diseases. They are not necessarily in the mainstream because going against the FDA and the establishment may get you ostracized by the medical community.

Some of the most highly educated people in our Ivy League schools won't even consider the possibility that there could be a brilliant alternative protocol that could heal diseases. I recently sat down to dinner with an Ivy League-educated, Wall Street executive who helps manage a $400 billion dollar endowment fund for one of the most prestigious universities in America. I told him my story of how I found a natural remedy for my daughter after she'd endured five years of treatment from a New York hospital. This gentleman gave me a condescending and doubtful look and said, "The last I checked, they had some of the brightest doctors in the world in that hospital."

"Yes," I said, with an equally condescending smile "and they could have killed my daughter if I'd listened to them. They're just not knowledgeable about anything except for what the AMA teaches them. In that regard, they are uneducated."

The Wall Street executive and I had a long conversation about my extensive research and the doctors I discovered. After hearing my explanations, he was more amenable to reading my book. If only American physicians were more open to using nutritional treatments in addition to their standard medical protocols. They're just too reliant on writing prescriptions instead of reading all types of research that's up and coming. Our American physicians need to reach out beyond what is printed in the periodicals that their superiors recommend. If they looked outside their closed circle and started reading reports by scientists who are presently working on new alternative discoveries in addition to the studies published by the AMA, they would learn more. They also need to look at the side effects of the new medicines that are being pushed by the big pharmaceutical companies. Doctors, I say, use your intellect and deductive reasoning powers BEFORE you push strong drugs on unsuspecting children and their trusting parents.

Here is what I suggest to the doctors: think before you write that prescription.

If you want to expand your knowledge and find a list of doctors in America who subscribe to alternative healing, you can go to my website and search for the physicians and others who have healed their patients and their families, not by using new, expensive prescription drugs but with alternative medicine.

As a mother and businesswoman, I want to analyze all my health and investment options. I invite you to do the same before you make a decision on how to heal yourself. My daughter is alive because of my tenacious research!

Here's how we saved her.

CHAPTER 1

Shocking News That Could Kill My Baby

"Courtney has autoimmune hepatitis #1," the doctor said with a grave look on his face.

"Autoimmune hepatitis?" I shouted back, trying to hold back my tears. "What is that? What does that mean? How did this happen?" The tears started to roll down my cheeks uncontrollably as Courtney, my beautiful, blue-eyed, seven-year-old daughter, just sat in the exam room and played with her new Groovy Girl doll, oblivious as to why Mommy was so sad and so mad at the new doctor.

Are you out of your freaking mind? I wanted to yell at this doctor. *You must be WRONG. How long have you been practicing medicine?* This is what I wanted to shout. I wanted to berate him and call him a quack.

Hepatitis? Isn't that a deadly disease? How can a little girl from the upper middle class suburbs of New Jersey get hepatitis? I was never an abusive drinker before or during pregnancy.

"Calm down Mrs. Otten," Dr. A. said quietly. (I'm changing his name and hospital so I don't have to hire a lawyer to deal with a disagreeable doctor.) "Let me explain. She has autoimmune hepatitis #1. It is not contagious. It's hepatitis A, B, and C that are contagious. She doesn't have A, B, or C."

So, I learned, she would be allowed to be around other children, and we wouldn't have to worry about any infectious disease. But that didn't make me feel any better.

"She will have to be on prednisone for a long time," he added.

That's when the panic set in and the tears started to well up in my eyes again. Taking prednisone meant serious side effects, IF it worked.

How can this be? I asked myself. I'm the most nutrition-conscious mother in my neighborhood. My three kids eat organic fruits and vegetables. I try not to give them McDonalds or Burger King or any other fast food, except for pizza. No sodas, no sugary breakfast cereals. And certainly no flu or pertussis shots.

What could I have done wrong for this to happen to my little girl? Sitting there in that doctor's exam room, I felt my life starting to crumble around me. I couldn't breathe.

The doctor continued. "She's going to have to be on prednisone and Imuran, an immune suppressant, for about five years."

I knew what that meant. I'd read about hepatitis. In fact, I'd worked next to a man with hepatitis C for years. He always looked like he was going to die from his interferon treatments. He also faced the possibility of a liver transplant.

The doctor had essentially just told me that *my gorgeous Courtney could die young*.

A mother's worst nightmare was coming true. And I didn't have my husband, Michael, there for support because I'd told him he didn't need to come to this doctor's appointment. I didn't think this appointment would bring such horrific news.

Now I had to repeat this diagnosis to my husband. Autoimmune hepatitis wasn't just a little virus she'd contracted. It was a death sentence. I dreaded going home to tell him. This was going to kill him.

CHAPTER 2

You Must Be a Quack!

It was talent show practice at the elementary school in April, 2003, when something happened that would change my life forever. My picture-perfect, affluent, suburban, working-mom life was shattered with the possibility of losing my seven-year old Courtney.

All the parents were happily watching their little stars practice their dancing and singing on stage when I noticed the whites of Courtney's eyes looked very yellow. This was easy to spot, as her eyes are as big and as blue as the Caribbean Sea. Since I was there with dozens of other moms, I turned to my friend Wendy Lynch, a nurse at the local hospital.

"What do you think of Courtney's yellow eyes?" I asked her.

"It looks like it could be jaundice," she said, "but I can't be sure. Better take her to the doctor tomorrow."

Having had experience with a jaundiced newborn baby, I wasn't scared or even concerned. In 1990, my first child, Adam, was born prematurely and weighed two pounds, fourteen ounces. The doctors told me that he just needed a good dose of vitamin D under the sunlamps and he would be better in no time. They were right. So now I thought, No worries. A little vitamin D and Courtney should be fine.

A week later, when the pediatrician checked her over, he looked very concerned. "I want to recommend a specialist," he told me. "She has jaundice, but I want to order some blood work. One of the best pediatric gastroenterologists practices in the vicinity. I would send my child to him."

He assured me that this specialist, Dr. A., was one of the best in this northern New Jersey hospital. I was a bit upset, but my pediatrician's faith in this doctor seemed genuine. The pediatrician had been a great diagnostician for the past thirteen years, so I trusted his judgment. He called and promptly got me an appointment.

We met with Dr. A., a pediatric gastroenterologist, the next week. He was also highly recommended by another mom in our town whose son had been treated by him for Crohn's disease. Dr. A. was a serious man who was also kind and very patient. I went to the appointment without my husband, Mike, who is always there for support, because I didn't think this appointment was serious enough to have him there. I said I'd handle it myself.

Dr. A. was a very slow talker, which was frustrating when my brain was formulating questions as fast as the hare was running in the race in the famous story, and he answered with the speed of the tortoise. The good doctor explained very methodically and carefully that my daughter had autoimmune hepatitis, which meant her liver was inflamed because her autoimmune system was unbalanced and not working, hence, her body was attacking her liver. Courtney would need treatment that would include prednisone to reduce the liver inflammation and later she would be put on Imuran (also known as MP6 or Azathioprine). Imuran would lower her immune system so her body would stop attacking itself and the liver would not get hepatitis (become inflamed). He would then monitor her every month with a blood test to make sure that she didn't develop cirrhosis of the liver.

Hepatitis? Cirrhosis of the liver? How did my seven-year-old contract hepatitis? When your blue-eyed, baby girl gets sick, and the doctor tells you it's her liver, you think, Oh My God. People don't live long, healthy lives with hepatitis. I've read medical articles that stated the patient can live as long as five to twenty years with a liver transplant. I was sure Courtney's life would be shortened. She might die young. Why Courtney? She's always been the happiest, easiest, and most beautiful child. My neighbor, Karin Barrett, used to call her my "Velcro kid" because she was stuck to my hip like Velcro. We were inseparable. We went everywhere together.

I couldn't stop crying, but I had to listen carefully to the doctor so I would understand the severity of Courtney's illness so I could repeat it to my husband.

The doctor's snaillike words were like a knife slowly digging into my soul. With every word he spoke, I felt as though my heart and stomach were being ripped out of my body. There has been no greater horror for me as a mother than when I heard that my daughter had autoimmune hepatitis. Not only did this disease have a possibly fatal outcome, but years later I found out that statistically only forty percent of the patients are actually healed by the standard, worldwide, medical protocol of prednisone and Imuran (or Azathioprine). The other sixty percent die early due to liver transplants or lack thereof.

The rest of my conversation with Dr. A. went by in a blur. I tried to control my crying as I asked as many questions as I could. Even though I was crying so hard I couldn't breathe, I kept telling myself I had to stop crying so I wouldn't scare my precious Courtney, who was sitting right beside me and playing with the doll she'd brought with her. But I just couldn't stop the tears from pouring out. It was that irrepressible crying that happens when you know you have no control over the situation and the possible death of your child is real. The thought that kept racing through my mind was that Courtney was going to die young and there was nothing I could do to save her. I've seen numerous movies in which the kid gets cancer or an incurable disease and dies young, but never in a million years did I think my life would turn into one of those tragic movies.

I finally regained my composure. Then another flood of questions ran through my head. How did Courtney contract this hepatitis? I'd heard it comes from alcohol abuse, but I wasn't a heavy drinker. I was the one in my large family that was always fit and trim and on what my relatives called a "nutrition kick." What was the success of the treatment Dr. A. was recommending? How long would Courtney have to be on prednisone? Would it get rid of the hepatitis forever, or would the disease come back? If the medicine did work, would Courtney be able to live a normal and long life? If the meds didn't work, at what age would she have to have a liver transplant? If she had a liver transplant as a child, how long would the new liver last? It's amazing how quickly your mind processes information when you're panicking, but I had to show the doctor that I was composed and patiently ask my questions and wait for him to answer them in his slow speech.

My idyllic family life was falling apart faster than I could imagine. All I could think of was, No, God—

this can't happen to my pure, innocent Courtney. She didn't do anything to deserve this diagnosis.

I quietly begged God to give me this disease, to take my arms and legs, but, please, God, don't take my daughter away from me. The tears started streaming down my face again.

By now, the doctor was trying to calm me down and assure me that he has worked with patients like Courtney for years. He looked at me with a straight face and said, "She should be fine in about five years with medical treatment."

I couldn't believe my ears. Five years on a pharmaceutical like prednisone? Are you f---ing kidding me? I wanted to scream. *She's just a baby! I've done everything I humanly can do to give her a healthy body. And this is the outcome?*

What had I done wrong?

True to my analytical nature, I continued my line of questioning. How many patients with this autoimmune disease that I've never heard of before had Dr. A. treated? What has his success rate been? What is his failure rate with these patients?

Dr. A. answered calmly that he'd worked with about two dozen patients over fifteen years.

That's less than two a year, was my immediate thought. That doesn't seem like a lot of experience with a life threatening illness. Maybe he doesn't know what he's talking about, I said to myself, and maybe he's got it all wrong. After all, he's a gastroenterologist, not a hepatologist. What does he know about long-term healing of the liver? And he could be a quack! He's had only two patients a year with this disease. Maybe because he's in the suburbs of New Jersey, he doesn't have enough experience. I hoped I would prove him wrong. I decided I'd better find a specialist in New York City. They always have the best of the best of everything in New York, or so it seems. Yes, I was ready to fire this quack on the spot. How dare he tell me that my seven-year-old has autoimmune hepatitis?

I needed a second opinion. Being a native New Yorker, I've always been a snob about New York having the very best in the world of everything. Surely I would be able to find the number one pediatric liver specialist in Manhattan. I also had to do more research to find out if this Dr. A. was the right doctor to use for this new-fangled autoimmune disease.

But in the meantime, he was all we had. According to this guy, we needed to follow his recommendation and to put her on high doses of prednisone immediately.

Even at that time, however, I knew that high doses of prednisone for several months caused puffiness, or "chipmunk cheeks," along with excessive hair growth. It can also cause diabetes. My poor, gorgeous, perfect girl was going to change into an overweight, hairy child who would most likely be teased unmercifully by the other kids at school. Then she would have to take another strange drug called Imuran, which would be the immune suppressant that was needed to prevent her body from attacking her liver.

I was devastated as I thought about the drugs I was forced to give my baby. It took all the strength I had to take the prescription from this Dr. A. and politely say, "Thank you for your help." When what I really wanted to say was, *Thanks for nothing you asshole. Thanks for the diagnosis that my daughter is going to die young.*

As we exited his office, however, I stayed calm and tightened my lips so I wouldn't start cursing him out. Holding Courtney's hand, I walked out of his office saying, "C'mon, sweetie, let's go get Daddy." Then when my sweet child asked why I was crying, I lied to her.

"Mommy, are you okay?"

I was choking on my tears while I replied, "Yes, sweetie. Everything's fine."

Everything wasn't fine. My seven-year old might die soon. *Hepatitis.* What have I done to her? The maternal guilt kicked in. It was unbearable. And, I was asking myself, how do I break the news to her loving daddy that his little Cordy Bear might not live long enough for us to see her go to college or dance at her wedding? How do I tell him that she might not live long enough to give us grandchildren? Worst of all, how do I tell him that the quality of her life will fall apart as her life is filled with drugs, operations, and more? What do I say to him?

CHAPTER 3

Giving up Control. How to Live With Autoimmune Hepatitis

When we got home, I told Mike what the doctor had said. He was as shocked as I was. But, unlike me, he didn't panic. Mike's a level-headed, analytical CPA. He trusted the judgment of the specialist and agreed with him that we should begin Courtney's treatment right away. Although I still had my gut-wrenching doubts about giving my daughter strong drugs, I had no experience or education in this subject, so I was forced to follow the doctor's orders. I prayed that the prednisone wouldn't affect her too much.

I was dead wrong.

I've been interested in nutrition since I was eighteen years old. As early as 1979, I started reading books and articles in periodicals written by many of the top nutritional gurus. This was before the Internet was invented. In the 1980s, I interviewed Shizuko Yamamoto for a college newspaper. She was the top person in NYC in macrobiotics. I've listened to Gary Null and followed the macrobiotic principles of Michio Kushi. I used the medical services of Dr. Ronald Hoffman for years and was introduced to homeopathic treatments by him. Now, with my daughter facing treatment by strong drugs and thanks to all this prior research, I had this overwhelming feeling that there must be some alternative treatment for AIH. After all, it was 2003, the new millennium! Now that I could turn to the Internet and the Yahoo and AOL search engines, I was sure there had to be someone on the World Wide Web who could help us. (Google was not well known in those days.)

In May, 2003, as soon as I got home from Dr. A.'s office, I got on the Internet and started my search for "nutritional remedies for autoimmune hepatitis." I found nothing but traditional drug treatments. I read online medical reports from Japan, Hungary, Germany, and the United States. Everything I read was depressing. The same protocol kept popping up. Prednisone and Imuran were the two standard drug treatments used throughout the world. And, the articles said, if the drugs didn't work, then a liver transplant would be the next step. A patient with a cirrhosed liver might die and their liver would have to be removed. Following a liver transplant, life expectancy was approximately five to twenty years.

The reports I read online cited many untimely deaths. The research and the deaths were documented in the research I found on www.pubmed.gov.

I cried myself to sleep that night. All I could think about was that this could be Courtney's life...a short, drug filled one. This was a real life nightmare. As I lay there in bed with my pillow wet with tears, this was the first time in my life that I wanted to die. I prayed for God to take me and to spare my daughter.

Within one month on the high doses of prednisone (30 milligrams for a 75-pound, seven-year-old body), the blood tests showed that as my daughter's liver levels were coming down immediately, her body began to swell up from water weight brought on by the drug. Dr. A. had explained that she would soon begin treatment with the Imuran, an immune suppressant, and when it finally kicked in then he would wean her off the prednisone. He estimated that she would be on the Imuran for about five years, or until her body reached its adult size, and then it would be okay on its own. I wasn't thrilled with the prospect of my baby girl on this medication for five years, but the idea that the treatment was "short term" gave me a bit of comfort.

Now that I had to capitulate and put my daughter on strong meds, I decided to renew my search for the most brilliant pediatric hepatologist on the East

Coast. It seemed logical to me that the very best and the brightest doctors would be working in New York City. We lived an hour from Manhattan, so I started searching there.

As luck would have it, one of the lacrosse coaches in our neighborhood was a doctor in the most prestigious children's hospital in New York City. We called him Dr. X. He claimed that his children's hospital was one of the best in the country. It had a superb reputation, and still does. So I begged him to find out who the pediatric hepatologists were and who had the best track record with AIH. Dr. X. was certain that the doctors he knew were the top specialists in their field. They had access to all the newest research and technology. After all, he said, a top Wall Street firm was their greatest benefactor and was pouring millions of dollars into the hospital.

Right away, I felt as if a great load had been lifted off my chest. I found a specialist in New York City. Dr. X. worked with this doctor and promised he'd get us an appointment with him immediately. I hugged Dr. X. long and hard right there on the lacrosse field. I truly believed Courtney was on her way to recovery.

It was not to be. This was the beginning of the worst five years of my daughter's life and the worst five years of my life, too. I was about to learn one of life's greatest lessons—even when the AMA and the FDA tell you otherwise, *trust your own intuition.*

It took us five years to learn about the brilliance, and the monumental flaws, inherent in the American medical community.

CHAPTER 4

The Best and the Brightest Doctors — NOT

Our first trip to the prestigious New York children's hospital recommended by Dr. X. was a success. (As before, I'm not naming the hospital because I enjoy the present state of my finances and don't want to be involved in litigation with a major institution.) Mike, Courtney, and I went as a united front to meet the brilliant New York pediatric hepatologist recommended by our friend, Dr. X. Mike and I were determined to find the best doctors to heal our baby. After all, a liver disease conjures up thoughts of hopelessness and life-long illness and, worst of all, an early death.

The next doctor we met with was Dr. Z., an intelligent, fast-thinking, fast-talking New Yorker with so much charisma and charm that all doctors should take lessons from him. His vast experience in hepatology and his complete knowledge of the autoimmune disease that Courtney had led me to believe he was the one who knew all there would be to know about AIH. Mike and I took to Dr. Z. immediately. Even though he was grossly out of shape, we both agreed he was brilliant. (I tried to look past his unhealthy physique because he was supposed to be the best in his field. Who am I to judge?)

So we instantly switched from the slow-talking New Jersey gastroenterologist to the more experienced, faster-talking hepatologist in the Big Apple. His waiting room was always packed with children with liver diseases. We were sure he was the one who would heal Courtney.

Even though Dr. Z.'s protocol for AIH was the same as Dr. A.'s, this New York specialist seemed to have more experience with this autoimmune deficiency. Liver disease was what he treated 24/7. He also told us that Courtney would probably need only about five years on the strong drugs that would suppress her immune system. When treatment began, she was seven years old, and by the time she would be about twelve years old and her body would be approximately adult size, the treatment would "kick in" and take care of itself. This gave us hope.

Nevertheless, Mike and I interrogated the doctor like we were Sherlock Holmes and Dr. Watson. Dr. Z. answered every question we shot at him with both speed and great scientific detail. He helped us to understand what our daughter's body was doing and how the drugs would help her heal. We grilled him for fifteen or twenty minutes. Mike, with his analytical accountant's intellect, and I, with my financial advisor and former journalistic skills, were a team to be reckoned with. We shot off so many questions that Dr. Z. looked exhausted at the end of our appointment. But what Courtney had was the type of case he dealt with on a daily basis. We felt he had the expertise that we needed.

But the biggest question, and the one the doctor never answered, was the one question most people probably don't ask when they get sick with an autoimmune disease. *How do we build her body back up to the healthy way it was before she got sick?*

That should be the ultimate goal! Another burning question: *If the Imuran or any other drug was going to "suppress" her immune system, then how was she going to fight off other viruses?* Wouldn't that mean that she would always have a compromised immune system if we were constantly suppressing it with drugs?

I'm no doctor, and I never wanted to take physics in high school or college, so I thought it just seemed illogical and downright stupid, as well as counterintuitive, that anyone should suppress an immune system for an extended period of time with powerful medications and then expect that the body would return to its healthful state without the assistance of supplements. I can understand suppressing the immune system for a short time to stop the immediate problem of jaundice. But stopping Courtney's body from attacking her liver was only a temporary solution, a Band-Aid, if you will. How would Courtney return to her former able-bodied self? I asked doctors that question for years, and every doctor danced around the issue.

Even Dr. Z. never answered that question to my satisfaction. He tried to convince me that it was *not important* to return her body back to "normal." What was imperative to him was to suppress the immune system *right now.* Within a month, the Imuran would stop her body from attacking her liver. And that was all he kept repeating. He was so convincing, and I was so confused and still so much in shock, that I just went along with the program. I gave up trying to get more information from him. He made me feel that he had all the answers. He convinced me that I shouldn't worry about anything. After all, I wasn't the doctor who had gone through med school and had fifteen years of experience with liver disease. This New York doctor was arguably one of the best pediatric hepatologists in one of the best children's hospitals on the East Coast. And me? I had no education in the sciences. My background was strictly business and journalism. So, I said to myself, he must be right. I'm only a financial advisor and a mom. I can help him with his investments and finances and cook him a healthy dinner, but I don't know medicine. So I must be wrong. Right? I should stop questioning his authority and sit back and be a good girl and follow the rules. Right? NOT!

This is how practically the whole world thinks. The doctor is right because he/she spent years in medical school and the patient didn't.

Like many parents, I was frozen with fear. Like a dumb cluck, I followed every word our specialist uttered. I was just happy that Courtney wasn't prescribed Interferon, which is given for hepatitis C (but not AIH). Back then, I didn't know a thing about treating AIH. In fact, I didn't even know this disease existed. So I followed the doctor's orders without question. This kind of brainwashing of patients like us by the medical community is prevalent in our health care system. They govern you by fear and control. But five years later, what seemed like inerrant mental persuasion would dramatically change into an intellectual battle between Dr. Z. and me. I no longer allow *anyone* to control my daughter's life using traditional medical protocols that don't make sense.

CHAPTER 5

The Prednisone Years

Prednisone is a vile drug. Sometimes, when it's an emergency or an acute illness, your body needs it immediately. But it can slowly kill you. I HATE PREDNISONE.

On June 23, 2003, when Courtney was seven years old, her aspartate aminotransferase (AST) and alanine aminotransferase (ALT) liver levels were 89/163. Normal AST and ALT liver levels are in the mid to low 20s. Her levels had come down a bit with 15 milligrams (mg.) of prednisone as she began her long, gut-wrenching journey on prescription drugs. The prednisone had now taken over Courtney's body...and her life.

In 2003 and 2004, her little 75-pound body was on 30 mg. of prednisone. At the same time, she was also taking Imuran and waiting for it to "kick in" and do its job of suppressing her immune system. During that time, her liver levels jumped to as high as 121/287 and fell as low as 25/34. It only took a couple months before she was ten pounds heavier. That was a huge increase for a genetically skinny kid. She also grew more hair on her body than some adult men have. During those years her arms had so much dark brown hair on them that some of the other kids at school called her a monkey. The excessive hair growth wasn't just on her arms, either; it was all over the body. When she was eight years old, her upper lip, eyebrows, and cheeks (sideburns) grew so much hair, she needed to use Nair. The constant teasing from children went on for five years. She also suffered from blood sugar problems, depression, and extreme weight gain. Her cheeks got so chubby so quickly that some of her classmates called her fat.

While these taunts tore my heart out, Courtney's inner confidence and wisdom grew. I believe there's a silent strength that many chronically ill children seem to develop that most adults don't muster up in a lifetime. With the unconditional love and support of her mom, her dad, her brother Adam, her sister Cara, and other close family and friends, Courtney found the words to fight back when the kids at school were so incredibly mean to her. Mike and I kept telling her it would only last for a little while, that she would be back to normal soon. She always believed her mom and dad. This must have given her some comfort.

I was proud of her resilience. On one occasion, a little boy teased her about having fat cheeks. What did she tell him? She said, "This weight is temporary and caused by a drug. But your face is permanent and won't ever go away." Her response may have been a little harsh, but she had to defend herself with whatever words she could. Whether it was thanks to the love of her family or the grace of God, she remained emotionally strong as she went through these tough times.

To this day, I still admire her confidence. My daughter was trapped inside an overweight, hairy body that she had no control over. But I could still see her beauty in her gorgeous blue eyes. Ironically, while her little body was puffing up, her aquamarine eyes were actually brighter than before because the prednisone made her cheeks pinker, and the contrast made her eyes stand out. Through it all, her spirit was never broken. Like almost any little kid, she continued to love dance classes and softball. Her friends' mothers were also so supportive of us during these trying years that I'll be forever grateful to them.

Another inconvenient side effect of his horrid drug was that it made Courtney have to get up to go to the bathroom in the middle of the night, every night. And she often wet her bed at night because of the water build-up from the prednisone. This made her afraid to sleep over at friends' houses in fear that she would pee in their beds. If she did have a sleepover, the wonderful mothers woke up with her in the middle of the night and guided her to and from the bathroom. Those moms knew her nighttime accidents were a result of that strong drug. They all felt so bad for her that they wanted to help her. Oh, those fabulous New Jersey mothers! (You know who you are.)

My poor, sweet baby also showed signs of a blood sugar imbalance. I wasn't sure if it was hypoglycemia or diabetes, but if Courtney didn't eat a full, healthy meal before bed, she would wake up at two a.m. screaming, "Mommy, mommy, I'm shaking." Since I have been hypoglycemic in the past, I realized it was probably her blood sugar. I would immediately run upstairs to her room with a plateful of food. I'm not sure whether her sugar was too low or too high because I never checked it at that moment. I was always too busy shoving fruit and protein into her mouth to stop her little body from trembling.

Eventually, these sugar imbalance episodes started occurring more frequently during the day while I was at work. Intuitively, Courtney always went for grapes or strawberries and stuffed them into her mouth to reduce the initial shaking, then she ate a healthy snack to make her body feel normal. When I did some more Internet research, I found out that one of the side effects of long term use of prednisone is diabetes. When I mentioned this to Dr. Z., he just said it was not related to the prednisone and I shouldn't worry.

Again, I couldn't believe what I was hearing. What I wanted to shout at him was *Are you f---ing kidding me? Do you think I'm an uneducated idiot and can't check the Internet? I wanted to say, Okay, let's say I was absolutely wrong about the onset of diabetes. Then why am I being woken up in the middle of the night with a kid who is shaking, only to be calmed down by immediately eating fruit followed by a complete meal at two a.m.? If it's not a blood sugar problem, then what is it?*

You would think the doctor should warn me about a possible sugar imbalance.

It was then that I realized I was dealing with someone who had limited knowledge of nutrition. I disregarded what he said, watched Courtney's diet, and made sure she ate a healthy dinner before bedtime. *I hate the side effects of prednisone.*

Each day, I reluctantly gave my daughter her 30 mgs. of prednisone, and each day I became more desperate for a cure, or at least an answer. She couldn't live like this forever! And if she didn't heal with this treatment of prednisone and Imuran, the next step was a liver transplant. I lived with that fear every day for five years. Courtney's persistent liver disease consumed our lives. Our whole family was exhausted.

The one silver lining was that through these tough prednisone years was that we felt great kindness and support from our neighbors and Courtney's friends and teachers at school. When she had to go into the hospital for a liver biopsy, her third grade teacher, the angelic Mrs. Manning, made all the children write get well notes. From September to June that year, Mrs. Manning and the other students watched Courtney change, saw the instant weight gain and extensive hair growth. Most of the other kids' parents explained that it was due to the medicine she needed to make her better. The biopsy would determine how much damage there was to her organ and tell us if she would be a candidate for a liver transplant.

Waiting for the prognosis was pure torture for all of us. In addition to her classmates making their own get well cards, Courtney's best friend, Kate Hearn, and her mom Ellen made her a balloon bouquet, and her Aunt Penelope sewed a beautiful, bright orange, heart pillow for her to hug at night and remind her that she was loved. Orange was Courtney's favorite color. Aunt Jackie had someone make a Disney Princess blanket for her.

The handmade card that really stole my heart was one made by one of Courtney's oldest friends on our block. This little neighbor boy never got along with Courtney, though they were classmates for years. He was one of those little boys who was so mean to Courtney and many other children, but, surprisingly, his card was the most loving of all. He cut a Christian cross out of brown construction paper so it looked like wood, pasted it in a card, and wrote "God Bless You, Get Well." As soon as I read the signature on this card, I started crying. This tough little guy was just as worried about Courtney as the rest of us. He didn't understand what was wrong and just saw that she looked puffy and different. He knew she was sick and had to go into the hospital for an operation so she couldn't go to school. You never know how loving kids are until one of their friends gets ill.

At the hospital that day, hours went by as we sat in the waiting room. When Courtney was taken from the operating room to the recovery room, she was crying, scared, and disoriented because she couldn't see her mommy and daddy. When they finally brought her to us, I breathed a sigh of relief. She was safe from the effects of being under anesthesia. But the suspense continued as we waited another few hours for the results of the liver biopsy. How damaged was her liver? Was she a transplant candidate?

The biopsy showed only slight damage to her liver. The doctor wasn't concerned. He believed the Imuran would work for her and that her liver should heal itself. The biopsy showed that she did not need a liver transplant. Thank God! Hopefully, Dr. Z. was right and she would never need a transplant in the future.

We would have to wait another four and a half years to find out that *he was wrong*. His medical protocol took four and a half years to fail.

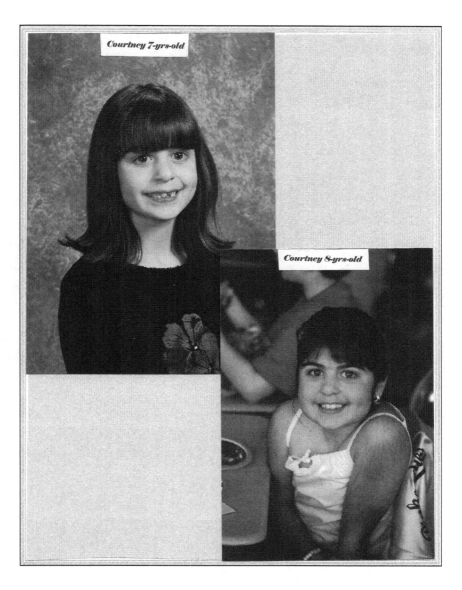

Courtney went from thin to puffy with prednisone

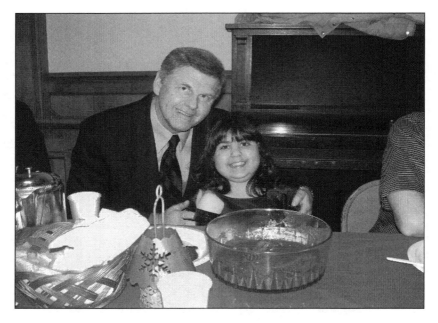

Courtney and her Dad

CHAPTER 6
Courtney's Courage

Every adoring parent thinks their child is the BEST in the world at everything. I'm one of those mothers who rave about their kids and love each of them more than anything else. My children are magnificent in their individual differences. My son Adam, for example, is a gifted classical singer and brilliant in science. My daughter Cara is a great athlete and a creative artist. But Courtney has a special gift that's served her well for almost a decade. That's *courage.* Besides the fact that she's an excellent student, gorgeous, and has always been a top athlete, her courage to stay positive in the face of this illness, which made her the butt of jokes in school and totally changed her life, is remarkable. She was forced to take drugs that made her young body swell up with water weight and grow excessive hair. She was often depressed because of the prednisone, and had to fight through the tears, puffy cheeks, hairy face and body, the onset of diabetes, and bedwetting. Yet through it all, she stayed sweet, kind, studious, and athletic. If I had to endure what she went through, I would have jumped off a bridge. Yes, I admit it—I'm not that strong.

One thing Courtney always knew was how much she was loved. Her confidence gave her the wisdom to shoot back verbal quips when nasty children made mean comments. From age seven to twelve, she obediently took her Imuran because Mom and Dad told her to. At the same time, she moved ahead in her dance class and performed at recitals. She had a voracious appetite for books and read every one her mommy bought for her. It gave her great joy to get lost in children's novels. But it was her passion for playing softball and watching Yankee baseball with her dad that raised her spirits more than anything else in the world. During these dreadful years, her dad became her best friend, and their connection has grown stronger and closer with each passing year. She went from being my "Velcro kid" to her daddy's best buddy. They watched New York Yankee games and USA Softball team games together and analyzed all the statistics for the Yankees and the USA Softball players. They even traveled to Oklahoma City to see the World Series of USA Softball. When they weren't at the ballgames, they laughed at their favorite G-rated comedies that included anything with Bill Murray and John Candy. They are still inseparable.

Courtney has taught the whole family to smile even when our lives looked like they were collapsing around us. If you just have the love and affection of your mom and dad, family and friends, she learned, you can get through anything. Or at least you can look at life and enjoy nearly every moment.

The liver biopsy in the fall of 2003 and the monthly check ups validated that the Imuran was working according to the standard protocol. Dr. Z. told us that Courtney was going to be weaned off prednisone and the Imuran would be all that she needed. *For now.* Following his instructions, we weaned her off the daily 30 mg. of prednisone and raised her Imuran to 100 mg. a day.

In just six months, she had gained ten pounds, going from eighty to ninety pounds, and now, as the prednisone was reduced, she started to slim down to her normal shape and size. She has always been a beautiful little girl, but having her body return to its natural state clearly made her a happier little girl, too.

But when the hair on her body didn't fall off, we chose to use Nair on the parts of her body that seemed to bother her the most, like the spaces above her lip and between her eyebrows. (She'd been calling that her unibrow.) In the summertime when she was nine, we also removed the hair on her legs so she wouldn't feel self-conscious in her bathing suit. She was on prednisone for fourteen months. We all hated what it did to her body and her emotions. She's always been a very smart child, at the top of her class, but because her body was changing so dramatically because of the strong drug, her emotions were often out of her control. She was weepy for no reason, and although we kept reminding her that "it's the drug talking," it was hard for her to stop crying. She was completely weaned off the prednisone in July of 2004, and she was thrilled at the thought that she never had to take it again. Or so we thought....

By May of 2004, her life seemed to be normal again. I saw Dr. Z. as my personal messiah. He had healed my baby. I hugged and kissed him in gratitude every time I saw him. I was in awe of him and this seemingly harmless drug, Imuran. *For two years,* Courtney and I went to the lab almost every month for her blood tests and to have the doctor evaluate her liver levels. She seemed to be doing better, but since her body was growing, we learned that she needed more medicine. In July 2004, her body was attacking her liver again and her AST/ALT liver levels went up again to 104/137. Dr. Z. told us that she needed to go back on the prednisone and increase her Imuran.

When she heard this, she started crying right there in the doctor's office. She didn't want to get fat and hairy again. She didn't want that body back.

She didn't want that awful life back. Mike and I promised to buy her lots of toys and presents to try to make her happier, but they didn't seem to help. Dr. Z. was very encouraging when he suggested that this would only be for a little while. I must admit that he was never an alarmist. He was always calm and upbeat, and his bedside manner was positive and supportive. It turned out that he was right; she only needed a few months on prednisone and then he weaned her off it again.

In 2005, when Courtney was ten years old, she was finally weaned off the prednisone completely and only on 125 mg of Imuran. It seemed as though the immunosuppressant was working. I was thrilled and amazed at the power of this wonder drug. Life seemed to be normal again, and our whole family was grateful. Mike continued his busy schedule as a CPA, and that summer I embarked on a new endeavor in a major Wall Street brokerage firm that required more of my time. This was at a time when our three kids were involved in team sports, homework, and Sunday Hebrew School.

By this time, I had accepted the traditional medical protocol and trusted the doctors blindly. I was so busy being a mom and a financial advisor that I stopped doing research on the Internet. What we were doing was the ONLY medical protocol I had found on the Web two years earlier. I focused now on building my business in this Wall Street firm and raising my children.

It wasn't until years later that I learned that Imuran was a precursor drug for leukemia. I learned that I had been willingly and unknowingly feeding my daughter a prescription for leukemia. This was an important fact that Dr. Z. failed to tell me until 2008. Another medical faux pas, in my opinion. If full disclosure is essential in Wall Street offices, shouldn't it also be mandatory in the doctor's office?

CHAPTER 7

Wall Street Hell While Raising a Sick Kid

How often does it happen on Wall Street and in corporate America that as soon as you switch companies for better opportunities, you discover that you've made a big mistake? In July, 2005, I was recruited by one of the most prestigious Wall Street firms. I thought I'd finally made it! I was at a top Wall Street firm, my baby girl seemed to be getting better, the Imuran was working. Life was great.

Then another bomb hit us. Five days after I was hired, my new manager was fired, and I was left to my own devices without the person who recruited me. I had no guidance or anyone watching my back. The next branch manager they hired made my life a living hell for the next two years. This guy was one of those standard Wall Street good old boys whose only concern was about climbing the corporate ladder. All he cared about was HIS financial success. So whichever male broker could help him make millions of dollars, that's the one he would favor and feed new accounts to, making that broker a million-dollar broker. The manager would prosper and look like a star, and they would both get big, fat, and wealthy, and to heck with everyone else. Sound like a familiar Wall Street story? In addition, it seemed that if you were a male and at the top of the Wall Street food chain, you received preferential treatment. But if you were a female and wanted to reach the top, then you'd better be a pushy broad or they'd run over you like a hot dog under a Mack truck.

Being a newly hired female in a Wall Street firm and trying to grow my business, puts me at the bottom of the food chain. And it wasn't a good place to be. During the next two years, I was subjected to so much discrimination and office politics that I had to watch my back all the time to make sure there were no knives in it. I thought that gender discrimination had been vanquished in the 1980s. Not so. It was still alive and powerful...only now, in the new millennium, they try to be covert about it.

If building my business in spite of having a cruel and malicious manager wasn't bad enough, Courtney's health also filled my thoughts. Was she going to get better after five years? Would the drugs work? In the back of my mind was this constant fear that she was going to die young. We know that liver transplants don't last long. My nerves were shot, on a daily basis. Some days I would have a great day opening up accounts and bringing in new business, and other days I'd be at my desk crying about possibly losing my little girl.

To make matters worse, one day in 2005 I overheard my selfish new manager telling his office buddy how he loved his dog more than he loved his two children. I'll never forget hearing him say, "I love my two daughters, but I love my dog more!" Whether it was in jest or not, that's when I knew I was in trouble. If he didn't love his own little daughters more than his pet, he probably wouldn't have much compassion for my Courtney's disease. But I had a five-year contract with the firm. I was forced to hang in there.

I kept my head down at work and tried to be "one of the guys." When I finally realized I couldn't penetrate the "boys club," I just focused on staying out of this manager's way. I kept focusing on my business and taking care of my kids. Keeping Courtney happy was my main objective, higher than anything else in my life.

A year later, near the end of 2006, the head honchos in this Wall Street firm finally figured out that my branch manager cared more about himself than keeping his sales force happy. Twenty-one brokers had left his branch because of him. They finally removed him from that management position. From that day on, I felt less threatened at work.

Now I could focus completely on my business and the health of my daughter without the distraction and fear that my manager was undermining me and trying to get me fired or in trouble.

During these two tumultuous years, I was so caught up in the dramas of office politics and not getting kicked out and trying to grow and survive in this Wall Street firm, I completely forgot to take Courtney to Dr. Z. for a checkup. It had been about eighteen months since we had last visited him. We were way overdue.

In the fall of 2005 after I joined the Wall Street firm, her liver levels were 44/56, which gave me a false sense of security that she was getting better on the Imuran. In February, 2007, I scheduled a blood test for her and a follow-up visit with Dr. Z. at the New York children's hospital. Once again, I thought that Mike would not have to come with us because for the past year and a half we thought Courtney was doing fine on 125 mg. of Imuran. She was her normal thin self again, and her eyes were not yellow with jaundice.

She had been off prednisone for about two years and the awful side effects—the prednisone plumpness, hairiness, irritability, and irregular blood sugar shakes—were gone. Courtney and I thought this would turn into a fun trip to New York City. We started out with our favorite breakfast at the local diner that we called the Shoebox Diner. It was a tiny, quaint diner that looked like a railroad car that served Courtney's favorite pancakes. We figured we'd run to the doctor's office after breakfast, he'd tell us everything was going according to plan and to stay on the Imuran for probably another year. We planned a girls' day out for lunch afterwards and maybe a little shopping in Manhattan to enjoy our special time alone.

The pancakes were the only good thing that day. Everything else turned out to be horrifying. Can you imagine how it feels when you're told that your child isn't doing well on the meds that were supposed to save her life? It was that morning when I found out that Courtney's life was truly in danger.

CHAPTER 8

A Mother's Worst Nightmare

As Courtney and I waited for our turn in the reception area in the pediatric liver wing of the children's hospital, we watched the sick children going in and out. All of them obviously had something wrong with their livers. Some of them were painfully sick with jaundice and prednisone puffiness. I remember sitting there with a heavy heart watching one beautiful young child in a wheelchair. This child, who seemed to be nine or ten years old, had a short haircut and was so overweight because of the prednisone that I couldn't tell if the child was a girl or a boy. How grateful to God I was that it wasn't my Courtney in that wheelchair! I was so happy that the Imuran was working for her. The tears were welling up in my eyes so much so that I had to turn away from this child and the mother so they wouldn't see me crying for them. You could tell that the child's future looked bleak.

When our turn came to go into the examination room, to my surprise, there was a new female doctor who said she was taking over some of Dr. Z'.s cases because he was swamped with post-liver transplant patients. While I'd become comfortable with Dr. Z., I was happy to see that it was a woman who was obviously Spanish and spoke with an accent. My family is from Puerto Rico so I'm always happy to see and be with Hispanic doctors. I feel a kinship with them right away.

But this woman was different. She was nothing like the charismatic Dr. Z. She was curt, rude, and void of compassion.

Courtney and I walked in with smiles. This new doctor sat us down and explained that she had been asked to help out today. She looked over Courtney's chart and the recent blood work, then started telling us, in her thick Spanish accent, that Courtney's liver levels were very high and we would have to put her on high doses of prednisone right away for quite some time. Her attitude was very negative, and she kept repeating, "This is bad. We need to put her on a high dose of prednisone immediately."

Courtney burst out crying. She put her head in her hands and then in her lap and was inconsolable.

I sat on the examination table next to her. Holding her head in my lap, I stroked her hair, and tried to comfort her. I looked at the doctor and said, "But she won't have to be on it too long, right?" I was nodding my head to give the doctor a signal to agree with me so Courtney would stop crying.

But she had her eyes fixed on the lab report and never looked at me. She kept saying, "This is very bad. We don't know, maybe a year, maybe two years on the prednisone."

Courtney was crying more than ever. I was ready to lunge at this ice-cold doctor and choke her to death. Every other word she uttered was so difficult to understand, because of her accent, that I wanted to scream, *Speak English woman! I can't understand half of what you're saying, and you're scaring my daughter! I'm going to strangle you if you don't shut up, you coldhearted witch!*

Even though I didn't actually yell this, I felt like my blood pressure was so high my body was going to explode. I tried to get her attention by looking straight at her with my eyes open as wide as possible and my lips pursed. If she could read my facial expressions, I thought, she'd shut up and stop making it worse. This insensitive, self-absorbed doctor was pissing me off!

Instead of losing my temper and punching her in the face, however, I demanded with an angry tone in my voice to speak to Dr. Z. and get a second opinion. She started to argue that he was too busy, but I gave her the "big eyes" again to show that I was dead serious. All this while my daughter was still crying in my lap. I insisted, with a voice that was just short of screaming, that I wouldn't leave the office without talking to MY DOCTOR. I strongly suggested that she call him right away because I wanted *him* to diagnose this blood work, *not her.*

She tried to calm me down, but I was furious with her horrible bedside manner and this killer disease. I felt like a lioness protecting her cub. I was ready to rip her throat out. My New York street kid was coming out, and I was using all my strength and will power to hold back my anger. I was sure she could see it in my eyes and hear it in my voice.

I was, in fact, mere seconds away from flying into a fit of rage. I'm not a very large person. I'm 5'7" and only 125 pounds, but at that moment, this doctor was causing my daughter such pain and anguish that I felt as big and as crazed as Mike Tyson. I could have bitten her ear off.

That's when I think she finally got it. She swiftly left the room and came back a few minutes later to inform me that we would have to wait a long while for Dr. Z.

I calmed down. "Fine," I said. "We have all day." I was exhausted from that nightmare called autoimmune hepatitis and I wanted it to end.

About twenty minutes later, Dr. Z. came into the examination room and with his always soothing voice started to explain that Courtney's liver levels had probably risen because she had grown in the last year and a half. She would need a small dose of prednisone, he said, to reduce her AST/ALT levels, which had spiked to an astronomical 258/429. He added that he would also raise the Imuran to 150 mg. per day and casually suggested that she wouldn't be on the "pred" for very long. He also insisted that we monitor her blood in two weeks and monthly thereafter.

Courtney stopped crying and sat up. His reassuring and comforting voice was making her feel better already.

My mind was racing with questions again. What else could they have missed? Why wasn't Courtney's body responding to the changes in medication? Why wasn't she getting better? It had been over four years! What was Dr. Z. doing wrong?

So I began asking him these questions. And more, too. I'm one of those people who are obsessed with nutrition and proper exercise. I've been interested in a nutritional way of life since I was a teenager and believe that good nutrition, supplements, and exercise are critical to maintaining a healthy body. Dr. Z. had been obese ever since we'd first met him, which now made me realize that maybe he didn't follow a healthy way of life. I don't want to imply that I'm judging him, or anyone else, who is overweight, but for several years I observed that he was not taking care of himself. That led me to believe that he didn't have extensive knowledge in nutrition, either. If he did, he probably would be more fit.

When I asked him, almost pleaded with him, if there were any vitamins that Courtney could take to help her body get back to its healthy state, he said, "No. She needs these meds." Then he said, "I don't believe in vitamins."

"Well, I do," I snapped back. Of course, in my head I was thinking, *Listen buddy, I've been the same weight for twenty-five years. You're clearly younger than me and obviously in poor health, so what's wrong with this picture??*

But he was the doctor, and we're all taught to believe that doctors are like God. We are not to question them. We should always trust them completely. Besides, I was never smart enough to get into medical school. I was just a financial advisor. I'm clearly not as smart as a doctor. Right? So he must be right. And I must be wrong. Boy, was I brainwashed.

After Dr. Z. and I sparred for another round or two, I backed off and stopped pushing the concept of vitamin therapy on him. Obviously, I was barking up the wrong tree. He was completely adamant in his opinion that vitamins don't work and that allopathic medicine is the only proper course of treatment. Even though I still felt in my gut that I was onto something, I knew I was not going to get any help from him with regard to nutrition and autoimmune hepatitis.

So, begrudgingly, I did what he suggested. After all, he had been right so far. But my confidence in him was starting to deteriorate. He had said that Courtney should be getting better within five years. She was well into her fourth year of treatment, and it didn't look to me like she was making progress.

Two weeks later, when Courtney was on 20 mg. of prednisone and 150 mg. of Imuran, her AST/ALT levels were 28/66. Lower, but still too high. Over the next four months as the doctor lowered her prednisone, Courtney's liver enzymes went down then jumped to 47/67. Dr. Z. then suggested the maximum amount of Imuran, 200 mg., while she was still on 12.5 mg. of prednisone. As usual, we went along with him.

At our next appointment, in June 2007, we learned that Courtney's liver levels were still not normal. Even with the maximum amount of Imuran, they were still high, 65/77.

Mike, Courtney and I went back to Dr. Z. and sat in his office as he calmly said, "Courtney's body is not responding to the Imuran and it's having a reverse effect on her. We want to put her on an alternative med. Cellcept. She has to stop the Imuran right away. We will keep her on the prednisone until we see her responding to the Cellcept."

The Imuran was not working! An "alternative med"? That's doctors' slang for a stronger and more powerful drug because your twelve-year-old is getting worse. We are not stupid parents. Mike and I are an educated couple and can read (and hear) between the lines. Dr. Z. was implying that Courtney could go on a liver transplant list if this "alternative med" didn't work.

My heart sank. I wanted to throw up. I wanted to choke him and scream, *What the f--k! You told me that she would be well in five years, and now you're telling me that she has to go on a stronger drug! When will this insanity end?*

I could feel that overwhelming putrid feeling in my stomach. Was my beautiful baby girl was going to die young? That's what you think when the doctor tells you the drugs you're giving your daughter are making her worse instead of healing her. I was beyond sad and scared. I felt hopeless and dumbstruck. Here we were at one of the best children's hospitals on the East Coast, and now this brilliant pediatric hepatologist is saying that the normal course of treatment has failed? And if Courtney doesn't take this Cellcept, then her liver will develop cirrhosis and eventually shut down? Or she will have to have a liver transplant? That her life will be cut short?

Mike, who is my emotional rock and my polar opposite, sat there in dead silence, though his face looked a little gray. I've only seen him look like that once before, and that was when our firstborn,

Adam, was not expected to live. At that time, the doctors told us that he might be born three months' premature and under two pounds and they would have to perform a C-section either tomorrow, next week or next month. We didn't know if Adam would live or die. We were encountering the same fear we were facing that day.

Mike and I were stunned with fear. Unbeknownst to me, Mike was feeling that we clearly had to do something different. This specialist and his protocol weren't working anymore.

As we sat there and digested what Dr. Z. was saying, my fear quickly changed to anger, then inquiry. The barrage of questions began again. Mike won't argue with a medical professional—he's too kind and is a big proponent of following rules—but me? I love to challenge and analyze everything. I need to know why things work the way they do. Or in this case, why this medical protocol failed.

I rarely back down from an intellectual fight. The main question I kept asking both pediatric specialists was never answered! And now it was my time to be pushy with Dr. Z.

"HOW," I began, "*how* do we get Courtney's cellular structure back to the way it was in 2002 before all this AIH occurred? She was healthy and well for the first seven years of her life. How do we get her body back to that level of health?"

What did the doctor reply? "We don't know what caused this," he said. "We just have to give her these drugs to suppress her immune system so it stops attacking the body, or in her case, the liver."

That wasn't an answer to my question!

My next (logical) question was, "If you suppress the immune system with these drugs, doesn't that make her more susceptible to catching viruses and colds? And won't that make her autoimmune system weaker? Which will then cause her liver levels to go up and cause more cirrhosis? And the vicious cycle will continue?"

"Yes," he said, "but she must have these drugs to suppress her immune system so it doesn't attack her liver and cause more hepatitis."

Oh. My. God. Now I wanted to smack him on the side of his head. He still was not answering my question. *What is this,* I was wondering, *a freaking joke? We're going around in circles like a dog chasing its tail!* I felt like Dr. Z. and I were Abbott and Costello, "Who's on first?" "I don't know." "Third base." Our conversation seemed that nonsensical, and it was then that I realized that I was getting nowhere with Dr. Z.

Yes, he was one of the best in his field. Yes, he practiced in one of the finest children's hospitals in the world. But here we were, going around and around with the same explanations and the same drug protocol, and my daughter still wasn't getting better. The only thing he knew was to use prednisone, Imuran and maybe Cellcept. (And any other drug that was FDA approved). After that, there would be a liver transplant.

What the heck? Did Dr. Z think I didn't have a brain in my head? It seemed to me that he was giving me the runaround because he didn't have any bullets left in his medical guns, and yet I was supposed to follow him like a lemming off a cliff!

No way was I taking this lying down. I was a New York Puerto Rican who was taught to fight for her rights no matter who put you down or told you that you didn't know what you were talking about. This was MY daughter, not his. And I wanted answers NOW.

My questions were answered with empty responses. The doctor had won this battle for now because I didn't have any research to support my idea that there MUST be another way to fight this autoimmune hepatitis instead of with these immune-suppressing drugs and liver transplants. I was beaten down. I was exhausted. I lost this round. When we left his office, Mike and I were both depressed and defeated. I felt like I'd gone fourteen rounds with Muhammad Ali and I'd lost in the fifteenth.

But Courtney hadn't understood the full meaning of our discussion with Dr. Z., though she had noticed that Daddy and Mommy weren't happy with the doctor.

Our ride home was sullen and silent. Both Mike and I tried to put on a good face for Courtney. We lied to her to make her feel upbeat and told her everything would be fine, we just had to get a different drug, and because she was such a brave girl, we would have to take her shopping for a gift. Now that she was almost a teenager, a doll wouldn't make her happy. So I promised to buy her some new clothes. Mall shopping! Of course, that did the trick.

We stopped at the drug store on the way home and filled the new prescription Dr. Z. had given us. When we got home, I was going to carefully read the warning label before I gave Courtney this new medicine. I didn't trust anyone anymore. I wanted to know everything about any pill I was putting into my daughter's body. Nobody cares more about my Cordy-Bear than me… except her Daddy.

That night, when only Mike and I were left at the dinner table, I picked up the package of Cellcept, opened it, and started reading the enclosures. The very first sentence said *Can cause lymphoma.*

That's where I stopped. I looked at Mike. I felt like I was about to choke on the food I was swallowing as I read the warning label. "Honey," I said, "we can't give this Cellcept to our daughter! This warning says 'can cause lymphoma.' I don't want to give her this. Do you?"

"No," he replied. I could hear the hopelessness in his voice. "But what are we going to do?"

Now my confusion turned to anger again. *This f---ing doctor was forcing me to choose between giving my daughter a drug that can cause cancer or let her die of a liver disease. And nothing else? What kind of screwed up society do we live in with medical advice like this? Are there no other choices?*

My reply to Mike must have sounded insane, but I saw no other way to go. "I don't know what we're going to give Courtney," I said defiantly, "but if I don't TRY to find a natural cure for my daughter and she dies from a liver transplant or gets cancer from this drug, I'll never forgive myself." He sort of nodded, and I went on. "I figure that since we didn't find Dr. Z. for three months when Courtney was sick in 2003, that should give me about three months to try to figure this out before she gets worse." I waited for him to say something, but he was still silent. "If I fail," I concluded, "then we will have to give her Cellcept."

Mike seemed to think it sounded logical. He knows that I love our kids more than my own life, that I would travel to the ends of the earth to save them if I had to. Because of my unconditional love and devotion for our daughter, Mike trusted my judgment...for now.

CHAPTER 9

Prednisone Puffiness for a Tween

During the summer of 2007 Courtney was on the prednisone again. And she was exhibiting all the horrible side effects again, too. She was puffy around the cheeks, excessive hair was growing all over her body, and she'd gained more weight around her middle, which made her feel fat. To top it off, her glucose levels rose to above 100 from time to time, and she exhibited signs of what I interpreted as borderline diabetes. Even if I were misinterpreting the blood sugar imbalance as diabetes, however, the lab work showed that her sugar levels were off and she was getting the "shakes" again, not only in the middle of the night, but often during the day, too.

Although I kept telling Dr. Z. that she was showing signs of diabetes or at least hypoglycemia and I thought it was from the prednisone, he denied that this was possible.

"No," he kept saying, "that's not the medicine. I don't know what it is, but I wouldn't worry about it."

I knew he was wrong, so instead of just arguing, I stopped asking and told Courtney we were going to make sure she ate three healthy meals a day and nutritious snacks in between so we could prevent the trembling. She became very aware of putting the right foods into her mouth and soon started to notice the correlation between eating well and not getting that shaky feeling.

Being an active tween, she was still obsessed with her favorite sport, softball. So one hot summer day we went to a poolside barbeque for her softball team and their families. Courtney didn't want to go because she would have to wear a bathing suit and all the other girls would see her hairy back and shoulders and her pudgy belly. I convinced her to wear a long sleeve T-shirt to cover up her hairy body and stomach. She begrudgingly said okay. But when we got to the barbeque and I saw her standing on the deck, looking hot and miserable but unwilling to go into the water because she didn't want her teammates to see how hairy she was. She was standing on the deck with her arms folded, fully clothed, in 90-degree heat, miserable and sweating, while her friends were splashing and having a great time in the pool. She looked so sad and angry. She just wanted to have fun and look like the other young girls in their bathing suits. Only Mike and I understood her emotional pre-teen struggle. So I tried to bribe her with twenty dollars if she would just jump in (wearing the long-sleeved T-shirt) and swim and have a good time with her teammates, who were trying to get her join them in the pool. Being a stubborn twelve-year old, she jumped in, hopped back out, and snapped the twenty-dollar bill out of my hands. She refused to stay in the water because everyone would see her fuzzy, pudgy body. As we had done before to make her feel like a normal young girl, we started using Nair on her forearms, shoulders, and back as well as on her upper lip, between her eyebrows, and on her legs.

These minor side effects may not seem like much to the average adult, but to a tween, trying to look like the other girls is critical to building self-esteem. My heart was heavy with guilt because I couldn't heal my own child. My husband and I never told Courtney, her siblings, her friends, or our family that she had a deadly disease. We NEVER wanted to utter the words "liver transplant," "shortened life span," or "early death," which are all possible if you are diagnosed with autoimmune hepatitis type 1 or autoimmune hepatitis type 2.

Autoimmune hepatitis type 1, which is what Courtney had, was explained by Dr. Z. as "better" than AIH type 2. While both types of AIH usually affect females (75 percent more than males), he said, AIH 2 is mainly a pediatric condition and afflicts infants and children up to about age of seven. Acute liver failure is more prevalent in AIH 2 than AIH 1.

CHAPTER 10

Searching for a Different Cure

It was in 2010 when we finally told Courtney how serious her disease was, but this was only after she had been well for three years. The power of belief is critical when you are healing. I read this twenty years ago in a life-changing book, *You Can Heal Your Life*, by Louise Hay, which my sister Michele recommended. Hay healed herself of cervical cancer with her positive affirmations, and her book documents her healing and gives details of the mental patterns associated with various physical ailments. Hay also developed positive thought processes for reversing disease and creating health in the body. She and many other New Age writers these days believe that the power of the mind can truly heal a person if their belief is strong enough. The medical community calls this the "placebo effect," but, simply put, the subconscious mind accepts whatever we choose to believe. I call it belief or faith in God. For those who are atheist or agnostic, I call it the power of their own belief.

After I read Louise Hay, I read *Love, Medicine and Miracles* by Dr. Bernie Siegel, a renowned surgeon who discusses what he learned about the importance of self-healing and the power of the mind. Siegel writes that "the mind and body are not separate units, but an integrated system." He teaches his cancer patients how a person acts and what we think, eat and feel are all important factors in healing your body. Love and unconditional belief are common themes in his books. Those who know the work of Deepak Chopra, an endocrinologist and author of at least a dozen books, understand what he writes about how our beliefs can dictate and are directly correlated to our health and wealth. Other authors who have written similar books are Dr. Wayne Dyer, Dr. Bruce H. Lipton, Gregg Braden, and the list goes on. One of favorite stories of belief and healing is from *Biology of Belief* by Dr. Bruce Lipton. He describes in scientific detail how your beliefs actually change the cellular structure in your body. I've also read how Dr. Bruce Moseley, an orthopedic surgeon and team doctor to the Houston Rockets, researched the specific benefits of arthroscopic surgery for arthritis of the knee. In his research group, he operated on ten middle-aged patients, five of whom received traditional knee surgery that included scraping and rinsing the knee joint or rinsing alone. The other five patients received a "placebo operation" in which Moseley simply made incisions on their knee to make it look real, then showed them a video of someone else's operation and told them they were watching their own operation live on camera. Six months later, all ten patients said they felt better and none were unhappy with their outcome. The "placebo" patients weren't told until two years later that they were part of the non surgical group. One of these patients was playing basketball with his grandson soon after the surgery. Dr. Moseley was amazed at the outcome and realized that it wasn't merely his skillful surgical techniques that healed his patients, but that their belief controlled their biology. Another amazing story of healing I read in Gregg Braden's book, *The Divine Matrix: Bridging Time, Space, Miracles, and Belief,* is about a young woman with an inoperable cancerous tumor who went to a medicineless hospital in Beijing, China. Because she firmly believed that the Chinese doctors could help, her tumor disappeared in only three minutes as her doctors gave her healing energy with their hands. She watched the miraculous shrinking of the tumor on a Doppler screen. (You can find this on YouTube.)

The stories in these books about self-healing were and still are motivational and uplifting to me. As a student of these teachings, I still believe it was imperative that we didn't tell Courtney (or anyone else) that her disease could have killed her if we couldn't find an answer. I recommend these books to anyone reading this. Some of these authors have been educated in Western medicine, and some follow the Eastern philosophies, but they all tell stories that will intrigue and inspire you to learn about the biology of belief and alternative healing. Read them yourself. Then you can decide for yourself which author you most resonate with.

In addition to the power of the mind, since 1978 I've also been a proponent of proper nutrition and natural healing. My grandparents came from Puerto Rico, where my great grandmother was called the town's "herb woman." According to my mother, back in the early 1900's people used to come to Great Grandma Christina when they were sick and she told them what herbs to take to heal themselves.

In the 1980s and 1990s, I found a community of people who believe many illnesses can be healed by holistic treatment. In 1985, I befriended a brilliant young doctor in New York who introduced me to the wonderful world of homeopathy and nutrition. This is Dr. Ronald Hoffman, who is now an author and the host of a nationally syndicated radio show called *Health Talk*. He treated me with homeopathic supplements and recommended certain vitamins and a healthier diet of no red meat, no white flour, plus vegetables and grains that I'd never heard of.

I later found books by Gary Null, Ph.D., and Dr. Michio Kushi, father of the macrobiotic diet.

I've always been an "outside-the-box" thinker, so when Courtney was diagnosed with this life-threatening disease in 2003, I got on the Internet right away and searched for anyone on the World Wide Web who had autoimmune hepatitis and healed themselves naturally or holistically. To my dismay, I found nothing and no one in the nutritional community on the Internet who was knowledgeable about the strange autoimmune disease afflicting my baby girl.

This was when I was referred to Dr. A. in New Jersey and Dr. Z. in New York. In 2003, these doctors seemed to be the only ones who could help Courtney. But in 2007 when Dr. Z. seemed to be telling Mike and me that if Courtney didn't take the alternative meds he prescribed, she might need a liver transplant, I went back on the Internet to see if I could find anyone whose AIH had been healed nutritionally.

For the next several weeks, I cried almost every day as I also prayed for God to give me an answer. I got on the Internet every day, searching for someone or something that had a natural remedy for AIH. I logged on in the early morning, in the afternoon at work, in the evening while cooking dinner, and again before bedtime. I was obsessed with finding an answer.

Adam, Cara, and Courtney were always finding me crying in front of my laptop in the kitchen. Adam once said he didn't know why I was always crying, but he suspected I was concealing the true severity of Courtney's illness. As an intelligent seventeen-year-old, he knew something must be gravely wrong for me to be crying so much. The kids kept trying to console me, and I always stopped crying and lied to them, saying, "Oh, it's nothing, don't worry about me, I'm just having a hormonal day."

I was driven like a madwoman to find a cure. I had to. Courtney's life depended on me!

CHAPTER 11
The Minister's Wife

In mid-June 2007, a small miracle happened when I found Ladonna's story on the Internet. After I read the story of Ladonna Jones, the wife of a Texas minister, I gasped and shouted to the whole family (and anyone else who might be within hearing) "I think I found it!" Ladonna's AIH went into remission with supplements, just a year earlier.

Oh, please, God, I said to myself, *let this be it.*

From that point on, I went with my gut and followed any and all hunches. Ladonna's website had no telephone number, so I had to send her an e-mail with my phone number and wait twenty-four hours until she called me back. That was probably the longest twenty-four hours of my life.

What did I learn from Ladonna's website? She told the story of how she holistically reversed not only the AIH, but also rheumatoid arthritis, diabetes, hypothyroidism, and depression. She was, she wrote, on her last leg, as her liver was 85 percent nonfunctioning and she was on the liver transplant list at a Texas hospital. She was an insulin-dependent diabetic whose blood platelet count had dropped below 70,000 platelets per microliter. (Normal platelet count should be between 150,000 and 450,000 per microliter.) She was clearly in far worse shape than Courtney was, and she was fifty years old. She was dying. A few years before, she had been on high doses of Imuran and prednisone and became so weak from her failing liver that she couldn't get off the couch. It seemed to me that her story could be Courtney's story, but more extreme.

Ladonna called the very next night. She has this soft Texas drawl, and she spoke very sweetly. The one thing that made this suspicious New Yorker skeptical was that she used the phrases "thank the Lord" and "God bless" in every other sentence she spoke as she described her health ordeal. I wondered if she might not be a holy roller with about as much credibility as Jim and Tammy Faye Bakker. Or was she unusually honest and reliable? Now I'm a native New Yorker. Even though I've been taught to be cynical and cautious, I tend to trust people when they are genuinely God-loving. And even though I'm Jewish and our religions are worlds apart, I felt a female kinship with Ladonna.

I was desperate for anyone to tell me something promising, and Ladonna seemed so kind that I took a leap of faith and trusted my intuition. Crisis serves not only as a powerful teacher but also as a catalyst for change. And at that point, we needed a BIG CHANGE for Courtney.

Ladonna's story goes back to July, 2004, when she was gravely ill with AIH, her liver was only functioning at 15 percent, and she was awaiting a liver transplant. As the wife of the minister of her church, she was well known and the parishioners all knew that her health was failing. One day in April, 2005, when she felt like she'd never get better, a man from her church suggested that she started taking a regimen that included glyconutrient-rich supplements along with a host of other vitamins. He said that he and others had been helped by these incredible supplements, which is called Ambrotose powder. He went on to describe how Ambrotose helps your body produce glutathione (remember that word!) to strengthen your immune system. Without proper amounts of glutatione in your cells, your autoimmune system works poorly.

In addition to the Ambrotose powder, Ladonna also found an endocrinologist in the next town who was well versed in nutrition and put her on a larger regimen of supplements. Mainstays of this protocol were alpha lipoic acid (ALA) and B-complex, which I soon found out also raise the body's glutathione levels.

Within one week of taking multiple supplements that included glyconutrients and ALA and going on a good clean diet, Ladonna was able to get off the couch. Two or three weeks later, she told me, she felt strong enough to go to church. About ten months later, in February, 2006, thanks to this extensive alternative protocol, her liver was 95 percent functional and she was off all medications. Now Ladonna sells those supplements and is a very active member of her church...and she's my own personal angel.

That June day in 2007, when I spoke with Ladonna for the first time, I kept saying to myself, *This is it! I just know it is!* I was crying and smiling at the same time as she told me her healing story. The more she kept saying how God helped her find the answer, the closer I felt I was to Courtney's answer. Call it crazy, but this Southern Christian communicated heart to heart to this New York Jew. We were speaking the same spiritual language. I knew in my gut (some say it's the solar plexus) that Ladonna had the answer I needed for my daughter. Later I realized she was my conduit to the doctors, research, and supplements we needed to heal Courtney's AIH.

Ladonna had created her website with the help of her husband Curtis, the minister of their church. This was way before Facebook and most of the other social networking sites, and so when I did a search for natural remedies for autoimmune hepatitis, her website was the only hit. Her website gave me hope that there could be an answer for my little girl.

After our thirty-minute conversation, I said, "Ladonna, send me all the supplements you think will help Courtney." When she told me the first batch of supplements would cost almost $400, I didn't hesitate.

"Send them next-day express," I told her. "Nothing is too expensive for my daughter's health. I'll pay for it."

Ladonna seemed very authentic to me with her Texas accent and her constant references to God. After talking briefly with her husband, she offered to personally pay the $35 it would cost to send the supplements next-day express. She trusted me to send her a personal check as soon as I received the package.

Wow! Here I was, wondering if I should trust *her*, and *she* was putting up $35 for me without knowing who I was. Something rang true for me when she did that. When was the last time you experienced that from a stranger? Ladonna then told me to call her any time and tell her about our progress, and she would help us in any way she could.

When I got off the phone after that first conversation and Mike came into the kitchen, I told him, "I think I may have found an answer, but it will cost us $400 for now and more later."

As you can imagine, he flipped his lid. "You don't know if she's a snake-oil salesman or if these supplements even will work!" he yelled. "Why would you spend $400 sight unseen?"

All of a sudden, I felt like a gullible fool. Had I made a hasty choice? A wrong choice? Admittedly, I was desperately searching for someone to help me heal Courtney. I'd been immediately sold on Ladonna's story. I stood there, confused, and listened to Mike rant and complain about my spending $400 without knowing a thing about this stranger named Ladonna in Texas.

Then he asked me, "How do you even know these supplements can help Courtney beat autoimmune hepatitis?"

As always, I took the argument personally. But when I was speaking with Ladonna on the phone, I'd felt a connection and a knowing in my gut that she was telling the truth. So I yelled back at my always logical husband, "I don't care if I have to spend *thousands* of dollars trying to find an answer! Say we spend $400 a month for one year…is your daughter's life worth $4800 to $5000?" I had been searching on the Internet day and night. I was furious at this awful disease that was killing my baby girl, and now I was angry at Mike and his skepticism. I screamed at him.

"This woman told me she reversed her autoimmune hepatitis with those supplements and nutrients," I yelled. "I'm willing to spend the money and take a chance if it can help save our daughter's life. *Aren't you?*"

Mike was speechless. He couldn't argue with that. Nothing is more important to him than our children. The greatest thing about my husband is his devotion to our kids. He would die for them...and so would I. We are crazy in love with our kids.

The money didn't matter, we finally agreed. We could always work a little harder and make more. I knew that's what Mike was thinking. But in all the world, there is only one blue-eyed Courtney, and that's our girl. You can't put a price tag on your kid's life. I didn't care how much Ladonna Jones was charging for those supplements. I was following my mother's intuition because I didn't have anything else, no one else to believe in. Ladonna was my only hope. The best doctors in New York had let me down after five years on their drug protocol. They had failed. They were FIRED. There was nowhere else to turn except to God and whoever God put in my path.

Yes, that's what I said. I believe God guided me to everyone who was able to help Courtney get well. You can call it the Law of Attraction, or luck, or energy, or anything else. I truly feel that because of my strong belief, desire, and prayer, I was guided to Ladonna by a higher power.

The next day I received my box of supplements and my Visa was charged $450. To my dismay, there was a thick brochure of sales materials enclosed, which encouraged me to start selling the supplements. My first thought was, was she just selling me these nutrients to make a big, fat commission? Was Mike right? Was she just a snake-oil salesman? Right then, I felt like such a fool. Maybe I was wrong. Maybe I was so terrified at the thought of losing Courtney that I couldn't think straight. A wave of anger rushed through my body, and I called Ladonna immediately and left a ranting, angry message on her voicemail. I was crying as I told her that I thought it was "inappropriate to send sales materials to someone who's trying to save her child's life." I left a long message. "I can't believe you sent these sales materials," I said. "I trusted you. If you're lying, I'll be so disappointed." Because she was a minister's wife, I didn't swear at her, but I was mad enough to. At the same time, I was hoping that I was dead wrong and Ladonna was as honest as she had seemed.

It wasn't thirty minutes before she called me back and started trying to calm me down and make me understand that the company always has her enclose those sales materials. She was not lying. She had been very sick and was on the liver transplant list with 85 percent of her liver not functioning. Many of these nutrients, plus other supplements, had saved her life.

But I couldn't stop shouting and accusing her of some wrong-doing. In yelling at her, actually, I was blaming everyone that I could think of because I was so scared my daughter would die. I was beyond hysterical.

Finally, her husband Curtis, the Christian minister, got on the phone and calmly reiterated that Ladonna was telling the truth. "She was near death," he said in his gentle Texas drawl. "She's our miracle story. These are some of the supplements that may help your daughter," he added.

I wanted to believe him, but Mike's words kept ringing in my head—*she could be a snake-oil salesman.* By that time, I was so confused and the thought of my Courtney getting cancer from Cellcept or undergoing a liver transplant was putting more pressure on me than I'd ever encountered in my life. I was cracking up. I was actually having a nervous breakdown right there on the phone with strangers from the South.

Curtis's voice was firm yet gentle as he said, "God gave us a miracle."

I finally calmed down enough to realize that this man of God was ministering to me right there on the phone. He just kept repeating, "God helped heal Ladonna," and his conviction which wasn't pushy or pious, made me feel like he was being genuine.

After listening to Curtis trying to be the voice of reason, I was finally calm enough to apologize and ask, "Okay, which supplements should I give her? And how much should I start with?"

Curtis put Ladonna back on the phone, and she gave me directions and recommendations, which I carefully wrote down.

After that long, tumultuous phone call, I called Ladonna just about every other day to get her help to fine tune what doses of which nutrients to give my little darling. Ladonna also provided plenty of scientific evidence that explained exactly how the nutrients worked.

Courtney's body was on the mend. Ladonna Jones is an extraordinary woman, a true Christian, helpful, loving, and very forgiving. We still keep in touch.

CHAPTER 12
Dr. Burt Berkson and Alpha Lipoic Acid

After two weeks on the nutrients I received from Ladonna, Courtney's blood work showed a slight improvement. I was cautiously elated. I wanted to believe we had the correct blend of supplements, so I asked Ladonna if she knew of any doctors that understood the benefits of supplements and had any alternative treatments for AIH. First she recommended that I read the research conducted by Dr. Reginald McDaniel on glyconutrients http://www.valdezlink.com/pages/molecularbiology-dietarysupplements.htm. After I read everything I could find, I wanted an appointment with him, but his office is in Plano, Texas, and he was always traveling and not easily accessible.

Next, Ladonna referred me to an M.D. in New Mexico who had completely rejuvenated the liver of a sixty-six-year-old patient with hepatitis who was close to death from a cirrhosed liver and was in the process of using alpha lipoic acid (ALA) and other supplements to help another young girl with AIH. This doctor is Burt Berkson. The young girl is Kortni Gehri. (I think it's a freaky coincidence that both girls are Courtneys...just spelled differently.) The woman Dr. Berkson brought back to health is Mary Joanna Bean. She's from Oklahoma. Her friends call her Jo Bean. I call her my other angel.

Kortni Gehri, who was a twenty-one year old, lives in California, and had ALT/AST liver levels that were as high as 222/232. She had refused standard medical treatment and opted to fly to New Mexico to be treated by Dr. Berkson and his intravenous ALA protocol. She spent two weeks at his clinic and felt much better with her liver levels lower from the treatment, but they were not in the optimum range of the low 20's yet. Ladonna gave me her cell phone number, and I called her right away. Kortni's mother, Susie, and I became fast friends. We had to. Our daughters were both sick with this horrid liver disease.

Kortni immediately emailed me about her experience at Dr. Berkson's clinic. She told me how his research and supplements seemed logical to her, as she had been brought up by a mother who was a nurse and had always believed in nutrition. Kortni also did her own independent research and introduced me to the work of Dr. Jordan Rubin and his book, *The Maker's Diet*.

When Jordan Rubin was in his twenties, he developed Crohn's disease, which is a type of inflammatory bowel disease. Even though his father was in the medical field, he couldn't find anyone who was able to heal him. At twenty-three years old, Dr. Rubin became so gravely ill with Crohn's colitis that his weight dropped from 180 pounds to 104 and he was 6'1" tall. Conventional medicine didn't work for him, but he refused to die. In his research, he discovered a diet of whole, living, enzyme- and probiotic-rich foods that, along with supplemental vitamins, helped him boost his immune system and reversed his life-threatening autoimmune disease. He turned his life around and earned his Ph.D. Today, Dr. Rubin owns a multi-million-dollar vitamin company and organic farm called Garden of Life. I was intrigued by Kortni's account of his journey and purchased his books the next day on the Internet.

Now I felt I was on the path! The doors of the nutritional community were starting to open up to me. Within just one week I had found two people who had reversed the illness from their autoimmune diseases after being close to death and another who was on the mend. I was on a roll. I was getting closer to the alternative answer for Courtney's disease.

In 2002, Jo Bean from Oklahoma, who is now seventy-seven years old, was given less than a year to live. She was so ill with hepatitis C that her oncologists in Oklahoma told her that she had two months to a year to live. She had probably had hepatitis C for twenty-five years, and her liver was now so extremely damaged that only one small part of the left lobe was still functioning. The doctors added that the only way she would live for perhaps a year was if she took the standard drug treatment, Interferon. After doing some research of her own and learning about the horrible side effects—and the great expense—of Interferon, she declined the doctors' recommendation. As Jo Bean puts it, "I prayed to God for the wisdom to know what to do." She decided to find a natural treatment, which was difficult in 2002. Jo Bean soon and "coincidentally" received a brochure in the mail from Dr. Julian Whitaker, a famous holistic doctor in California. This brochure contained an article describing Dr. Burt Berkson's treatment of hepatitis C with ALA and low-dose naltrexone.

She immediately purchased Berkson's book, *The Alpha Lipoic Acid Breakthrough: The Superb Antioxidant That May Slow Aging, Repair Liver Damage, and Reduce the Risk of Cancer, Heart Disease, and Diabetes*. She read it twice. Then she phoned Dr. Berkson to schedule an appointment. He had a long waiting list, but the nurses squeezed Jo in right away. Jo and her husband, Lavan, drove 700 miles from Oklahoma to Las Cruces, New Mexico, for her first appointment. In December, 2002, when she walked into Dr. Berkson's clinic for the first time, she weighed about seventy-five pounds and, she says, "I was skin and bones. By then, I was so weak I couldn't even raise my arm to brush my hair." Her hepatitis C was so advanced that she could barely speak above a whisper. Her husband practically carried her into the doctor's office.

Dr. Berkson immediately began treatment. After the two weeks of intravenous antioxidant treatments, a strict change of diet, and supplemental vitamins, when Jo Bean went home to Oklahoma, she was strong enough to clean her 2000-square-foot house from top to bottom. This was something she had been unable to do for a year. She returned to the clinic every quarter in 2003 for more treatments. In fact, she felt so energized that she began driving by herself to Dr. Berkson's Las Cruces clinic. Her liver levels were steadily improving, and only four months later, an MRI and lab tests revealed that her liver was almost completely rebuilt and she was in remission. It's been ten years since Jo Bean met Dr. Berkson. Now she travels back annually for her IV treatment. Today she is a strong, happy grandmother who takes care of everything in her house. She later took care of her ailing husband until he passed away. Her case is another witness to the benefits of alternative treatments with ALA.

Dr. Burt Berkson's practice in Las Cruces, New Mexico, has been very successful in treating autoimmune diseases with intravenous ALA, B-complex, low-dose naltrexone, silymarin, and several other supplements. He has also had success treating multiple sclerosis, COPD, and some forms of cancer, including pancreatic cancer, with his antioxidant protocol. He has written four books on nutrition and healing.

Ladonna gave me Jo Bean's e-mail address and we soon became pen pals. After reading her amazing life story, I immediately called Dr. Berkson's office and spoke with his most trusted and kindest employee, his wife Ann. (She just happened to answer the phone that day.) I explained my dilemma and the five-year ordeal Courtney had endured and said that now her doctor had prescribed Cellcept. I begged Ann to have Dr. Berkson see my daughter right away because I didn't think we had much time before her liver levels would start to rise into the hundreds again.

Ann was gentle and understanding, but she explained that they couldn't accept pediatric patients because the doctor was not a board-certified pediatrician. She referred me to a pediatrician located near the Cleveland Clinic in Ohio who uses a similar protocol, but I begged her to at least *consider* my daughter as a patient as she was not getting better on the traditional medical treatment, and the alternative leukemia drug was not a positive alternative. Ann was very empathetic as she lovingly explained that they are not experienced with children. She strongly recommended that I call the doctor in Cleveland.

I was dumbstruck at her rejection. How could any doctor's office turn down my poor daughter?

But Ann Berkson was extraordinarily kind, and I did understand her position. They just couldn't take on the responsibility of a pediatric patient. In recommending the doctor in Ohio, she was doing the only other thing she could do to help me. The problem was that I didn't know anyone who had been to this Ohio doctor. Dr. Berkson was the man who helped Jo Bean's Hepatitis C go into remission after her doctors gave her less than a year to live. Jo was a walking billboard for the Berkson clinic. Now he was treating Kortni Gehri. If Dr. Berkson could reverse the cirrhosis of a sixty-six-year-old woman who was close to death, surely he should be able to help a far healthier, younger body with a similar disease. I wanted HIM and no one else!

So I did what any committed and desperate mother would do: I copied his alternative protocol exactly and gave my Courtney all the supplements that Jo Bean and Kortni Gehri had received when they were sent home after Dr. Berkson's two-week treatment. The only thing I couldn't buy was the low-dose naltrexone (LDN), which I needed a prescription for and a doctor to monitor it. I purchased all the other vitamins and nutraceuticals from the same company that Dr. Berkson used at the time and prayed that Courtney wouldn't need the LDN.

But there was still a key ingredient missing. I needed an M.D. to guide me and read Courtney's blood test results. I wanted to work with a doctor who could validate that what I was doing was the right thing. I'm like a pit-bull when I want something badly enough. I wanted to save Courtney's life.

With these two stories of complete and partial remission, I knew I'd found my doctor and the answer to this deadly disease. I was sure the answer was with Dr. Burt Berkson. My research on him proved that he was not only an independent thinker, but he had also earned a Ph.D. before he acquired his M.D. This means he was trained as a scientist trying to discover answers via deductive reasoning in a laboratory instead of simply memorizing drug treatments from textbooks.

While medical doctors are taught to retain an extraordinary amount of information and diagnose a patient as accurately as possible, they are only schooled in one direction. That is Western medicine. Admittedly, students who are accepted into and graduate from medical schools are often some of the most brilliant people in the world. The problem remains, however, that this intellectual breed is specifically instructed to follow the FDA guidelines that the AMA dictates. If they ask difficult questions, if they attempt to step out of line merely because they think that it might be beneficial to the patient to do something, say, alternative, they can be fined or lose the license they've worked so hard to earn. I understand that we need rules and regulations and that the medical profession needs to be monitored so doctors don't overdose their patients. But the narrow-mindedness of the AMA leaves little room for truly independent thinkers. There are at least four other popular modes of holistic nutrition that have successfully been used by doctors worldwide. But these modes are not incorporated into our standard American medical practice.

For centuries, European doctors have been schooled in homeopathy. Eastern and some Western doctors use Chinese herbs. In India, Ayurvedic medicine is common. And let's not forget the science of vitamins and nutraceuticals that is relatively new in America. Why do we not teach our medical professionals to incorporate these ancient and new technologies into their medical protocols? One answer that's been whispered throughout the decades is that holistic remedies do not financially benefit the American pharmaceutical industry.

While many lives are saved by new drugs discovered in Big Pharma's laboratories, it is these same pharmaceutical companies that fund the medical schools with millions of dollars and their own brands of medicine. The FDA is swayed by the pharmaceutical companies to approve certain drugs. If a new drug is not very profitable for Big Pharma, then it's likely that they won't be motivated to put it on the market. They don't have any reason to push it through the FDA for approval. It's a vicious cycle that's controlled and dictated by the greed of the pharmaceutical industry. For example, ALA research was shut down by the FDA, even though it is known to regenerate the liver and aid in reversing diabetes, multiple sclerosis, and other autoimmune diseases.

This is where Dr. Burt Berkson is a cut above the rest. While studying for his Ph.D., he was trained by his professors to "prove them wrong." As a scientist, he was taught to always ask questions. That's my kind of analytical thinker!

After I read all about Dr. Berkson, my logical, financial brain kicked in. I started wondering how much it would actually cost us if the worst-case scenario happened and Courtney did have to have a liver transplant. The supplements were pricey, but when you compare them to the cost of a liver transplant, the vitamins and nutraceuticals are unbelievably affordable! According to the information I found on the Internet, the average total charge per transplant is approximately $577,100. This includes, they say, "30 Days Pre-transplant, Procurement of a liver from a donor, Hospital Transplant Admission, Physician During Transplant, 180 Days Post-transplant Admission, and Immunosuppressants." This is a great business for doctors who perform transplants! It is financially better than administering alternative nutritional therapy that could be validated scientifically. In 2007, the cost of Dr. Berkson's treatment was only $3,000 for the two weeks in Las Cruces, plus supplements and nutraceuticals to take home at the tune of approximately $400 a month. If half of the liver transplant and hepatitis C patients found someone like Dr. Berkson in every hospital in America, the liver transplant industry would lose billions of dollars. This protocol has also been able to help diabetes, multiple sclerosis, COPD, and some cancers. Imagine if it was embraced by the FDA. The Mayo Clinic could conceivably go out of business! That's why there's no motivating factor to teach doctors about ALA and LDN and other non-AMA treatments and medicines.

I felt that I'd found the answers for Courtney with Dr. Berkson's protocol. But I was still swimming alone in this ocean of alternative healing without a lifeguard watching over me. I was following my new friends who were patients being guided by their doctors. Even though my posse of ladies around the country was supporting me on a daily basis, I had to rely on my own maternal instincts to make sure Courtney was getting the right cocktail of supplements. My search continued for another doctor to help me tweak these supplements if necessary.

I was still using Dr. Z. to help me read the results of the bi-monthly blood work, but he would be useless in helping determine if the alternative protocol was working. He probably thought I was crazy, anyway, and was most likely waiting for me to come running back to him for help and more prednisone and Cellcept.

While Dr. Z. was arguably one of the most brilliant hepatologists in the tri-state area (New York, New Jersey, Connecticut), he had little experience or knowledge in the field of nutrition. I was on my own to figure it all out. Frankly, I was scared.

CHAPTER 13

Gluta-what? Glutathione Explained

In one of my weekly phone calls to Ladonna, I asked her if there were any more doctors in the northeast that I could contact who have had success with children and improving their autoimmune system with nutrition. I wasn't completely sold on this multi-level marketing product I'd bought from her, even though it was filled with host of natural, harmless ingredients, along with amino acids and minerals that Courtney wasn't getting in her daily food intake. I knew Ladonna's health had been completely restored by a combination of supplements, I was still doubtful. You must understand how tough it is to try to save your baby's life with an alternative answer when the rest of the world tells you you're crazy, you're wrong, you'll never find the answer. Almost everyone told me to listen to the doctor at the famous New York children's hospital. Even some of the top executives at the brokerage firm where I worked advised me that the pediatric physicians in this hospital were the very best in New York City. After all, my company was one of the largest benefactors to that hospital and was expanding their pediatric wing.

Being on the computer day and night and researching the benefits of raising your glutathione level with vitamins and nutraceuticals was a daunting task. Being a financial advisor in a major Wall Street brokerage firm, I was already on memory overload with financial data. Adding to that, I was scouring the Internet for ways to heal Courtney, plus carrying out my maternal responsibilities to my other two children and my husband. Now I needed to find an M.D. who would tell me, "Yes, you're doing the right thing. There are other children who have been healed of AIH with this antioxidant protocol."

Courtney had been on the supplements for only a few weeks. I needed to see more improvement more quickly to validate this new path we were on.

You have to understand this about me. While I was growing up in Queens, New York, in a middle-income household, I never strayed far from tradition. While I was the "good" kid who tried to follow the rules, I also tended to question everything. In high school and college, I kept getting into trouble for asking too many questions. In the business world, I challenged my bosses. Some people, in fact, found me a bit confrontational because I was always disagreeing with the standard procedures and protocols. I've never been a maverick, however, and always seemed to follow the other baby boomers. We're a generation famous for asking questions.

So walking this path alone was very scary for me. But no matter what, *I had to save my kid's life.*

Around the same time I started researching Dr. Berkson and his successes, Ladonna recommended that I speak to Dr. Emil Mondoa, a pediatrician who wrote *Sugars That Heal: The New Healing Science of Glyconutrients.*

Oh My God, I thought. A doctor who wrote a book on the subject! And he's a board certified pediatrician! Surely he'll know about children who have been helped with glutathione boosting nutrients.

But what were these *gly-co-nutrients* that Ladonna kept talking about? Here's what I learned. Glyconutrition, in layman's terms, is the science that improves your cellular structure and boosts the *glutathione* levels in your cells so your body can heal and boost its own immune system. According to several reports I read in 2007, the nutrients Ladonna introduced me to may help our cells produce their own glutathione.

That was another term I had to become familiar with. What is glutathione? It's a tripeptide, or protein made up of three different amino acids in each cell of our body, which are gamma-glutamic acid, cysteine, and glycine. Glutathione is a nutrient that is produced within our cells that forms enzymes such as glutathione peroxidase, which is essential to life. It's a potent antioxidant nutrient and a powerful scavenger of free radicals. It also detoxifies the cells by pulling chemicals, pollutants, and toxins out of them. According to the mountains of research on glutathione and auto-immune diseases I did, your body must produce the proper glutathione level in order to have a balanced immune system. This was more information I had to digest in addition to the enormous amount of data I had already read.

Since I started researching glutathione (GSH) in 2007, I've learned that there are multitudes of vitamins, nutraceuticals and super foods that help the body produce it. It seems that everywhere I go now and share my story of healing Courtney and raising the body's GSH level, I find another person selling a supplement that supposedly does the same thing. But the nutritional protocol that Ladonna and Jo Bean used were the only ones that I found at that time, so I followed their lead.

Ladonna suggested that I read Dr. Emil Mondoa's book because he had researched the benefits of glyconutrients. She also encouraged me to contact him if I had questions about the benefits of these nutrients. I Googled Dr. Mondoa right away and found out that he worked in southern New Jersey. Eureka! More help and more hope!

In August, 2007, when we took our annual family vacation on Long Beach Island, New Jersey, I read Dr. Mondoa's book from cover to cover. If he had an answer for Courtney, I wanted it fast. As I read the book, I also cross-referenced information I found on the Internet about GSH. Here's an excerpt from a published report in 2004 of how glutathione repairs the body, according to the University of Arkansas for Medical Sciences and their Department of Pediatrics:

"Glutathione protects cells in several ways. It neutralizes oxygen molecules before they can harm cells. Together with selenium, it forms the enzyme glutathione peroxidase, which neutralizes hydrogen peroxide. It is also a component of another antioxidant enzyme, glutathione-S-transferase, which is a broad-spectrum liver-detoxifying enzyme. Glutathione protects not only individual cells but also the tissues of the arteries, brain, heart, immune cells, kidneys, lenses of the eyes, liver, lungs, and skin against oxidant damage. It plays a role in preventing cancer, especially liver cancer, and may also have an anti-aging effect. Glutathione can be taken in supplement form. The production of glutathione by the body can be boosted by taking supplemental N-acetylcysteine or L-cysteine plus L-methionine. Studies suggest that this may be a better way of raising glutathione levels than taking glutathione itself. Glutathione is not technically an amino acid, however, due to its close relationship is normally grouped with the amino acids. Most glutathione is found in the liver where it detoxifies many harmful compounds to be excreted thru the bile. Some glutathione is released directly by the liver into the bloodstream where it helps to maintain the strength of your red blood cells and also protecting your white blood cells. Glutathione can also be found in the lungs and in your body's intestinal tract system. It is required for carbohydrate metabolism. Glutathione also appears to have anti-aging effects by aiding in the breakdown of oxidized fats that may contribute to atherosclerosis. As we get older glutathione levels in the body get lower and this can cause an increase in the aging process. Thus glutathione supplementation is useful to prevent this from occurring."[1]

All the cross referencing that I did on the Internet made me a believer. These supplements made sense. I read excerpts from Dr. Mondoa's book to Mike so he could understand why I was pumping Courtney so full of all these supplements. As soon as I finished the book, I told him I wanted to make an appointment with Dr. Mondoa and that I wanted him to come with us. I wasn't going to go through a new appointment alone again. I needed emotional

1   http://www.tacanow.org/family-resources/detoxification-glutathione-autism/ (accessed 1/8/08)

support. Mike needed emotional support, too. We were both scared to death that Courtney might die young. That's what might have happened if she'd had a liver transplant in 2007.

After returning home from our vacation, I tracked Dr. Mondoa down and begged him to meet with us. He admitted that while he'd had much success with the glyconutrients and some autoimmune diseases, he hadn't had any experience with AIH. But he was confident that the nutrients should help Courtney's body in some way. I didn't know how much he could contribute to my crusade to save my daughter's life, but I was desperate for validation from a pediatrician who had been successful with an alternative therapy.

Dr. Mondoa is a tall, soft-spoken man. When we went to his office for our first appointment, he examined Courtney and said he was surprised to see that she looked healthier than the blood work indicated. He expressed his interest in following her case and gave me his cell phone in case I needed to ask him any questions. He wanted to help, in any way he could. Our two-hour trip to visit Dr. Mondoa seemed like a waste of time to Mike and Courtney, but I received the intellectual support I needed to keep going along our nutritional path.

Now I looked at my resources. I had Dr. Burt Berkson's extensive antioxidant protocol to follow. He had reversed the cirrhosis of Jo Bean's hepatitis

C, plus Jo knew several other patients of Dr. Berkson who were successfully treated for autoimmune diseases. (Because of confidentiality issues, however, I wasn't privy to their names and phone numbers, but since Jo has been going to Berkson's office for ten years for annual treatments, she's made a scrapbook photo album of those patients whose autoimmune disease or other illness is in remission because of him and she's befriended many of them.) There was also my new buddy, Kortni Gehri, who was on the mend, even though she'd only had one treatment by Dr. Berkson. Also, I had met with Dr. Mondoa. Now I desperately wanted to find a doctor that I could meet on the East Coast who had reversed the symptoms of AIH naturally.

Yes, by mid-August, 2007, I was feeling much more confidence in the nutritional protocol I had pieced together. Even though Courtney's liver levels were relatively high while she was still on 10 mg. of prednisone, her AST/ALT never went above 74/88. This was somewhat encouraging because her liver enzymes hadn't risen to triple digits as they had in the past. They seemed to be leveling off.

But my time to reverse her cirrhosis was running out. I needed a miracle, *and fast.*

CHAPTER 14

Dr. Douglas Willen and Food Allergies

When I phoned Ladonna after we came home from our vacation, she also remembered that there was a reputable New York chiropractor who recommended vitamin supplements to his patients who had autoimmune diseases. This was Dr. Douglas Willen, who ran the Willen Wellness Center in New York City and had successfully helped patients with AIH.

I felt like I'd won the lottery. I was sure Dr. Willen was someone who obviously knew about holistic nutrition, as he had a thriving practice in Manhattan, home to eight million people. I wanted to meet with him right away, but he was extremely busy with speaking engagements and his practice in New York. Then I learned that he lived in central New Jersey, not far from our home. I phoned him and begged him to please see Courtney immediately, as I was running out of time to heal her. When I explained my hypothetical timeline of three months, he agreed to see us at his home.

We drove to his home the very next day. Courtney wasn't crazy about meeting yet another doctor, but this guy added something different to the mix. He encouraged me to give her the alpha lipoic acid, silymarin, selenium, and the other nutrients she was already on (thanks to Ladonna). He said he had also had success with them. But he was adamant that we needed to find out what foods she was allergic to and introduce a clean, alkaline diet.

This made perfect sense to me, as my other daughter, Cara, has extreme food allergies that give her horrible eczema and asthma. She has to maintain an alkaline diet and we've eliminated the foods she's allergic to in order to clear up the skin disorder.

I had an *aha!* moment in Dr. Willen's home office. Cara's extreme food allergies, eczema, and asthma were also autoimmune related! Courtney's AIH was just another manifestation of a body suffering from an imbalanced immune system that needed adjusting. When I asked Dr. Willen if I was correct, he said yes, adding that he was pleased that I had made that connection.

When we arrived, Dr. Willen's wife had greeted us warmly at the front door and immediately tried to comfort me by reiterating that her husband has had great success with helping patients with autoimmune diseases. Then Dr. Willen had walked out of his home office, and I was instantly in awe of his physical appearance. He has a very handsome face and is obviously someone who takes pride in his physique. You can tell that he works out. He was and still is the epitome of health. And his bedside manner is outstanding. He makes you feel empowered with all the information he offers you and the books he wants you to read.

This doctor also practices the fundamentals of nutrition at home and has his own children on a high-vitamin regimen. On a physical and holistic level, Dr. Willen was the antithesis of Dr. Z. at the famous New York children's hospital. Although they are about the same age and both are committed to their patients, one practices basic nutritional dietary principles daily, whereas the other didn't have a clue as to how to implement them into his life. Dr. Willen also does not talk down to his patients.

He said that Courtney needed to balance her immune system before it destroyed her liver completely and added that he would help me strengthen and support her body by introducing a variety of glutathione-raising supplements, along with a major dietary change. He suggested that Courtney might be allergic to the foods she was eating (which I already knew was true) and said she could also be suffering from "leaky gut syndrome." I had never considered that food allergies might be partly responsible for autoimmune diseases. Even though I had read most of *The Maker's Diet* by Jordan Rubin and Charles F. Stanley, I hadn't thought it would apply to AIH.

I knew, as soon as he started talking about "leaky-gut," kinesiology, probiotics, and ALA, that this was my guy. He also recommended several books for me to read so that I could educate myself further. (I had already read or heard about half the books he suggested.) Dr. Willen was the last piece I was looking for to solve the puzzle of my daughter's disease. Even though he's a chiropractor and not an M.D. like Burt Berkson, he was using a similar health-creating protocol.

The concept of food allergies was something I'd never considered before, but one of the reasons I listened to Dr. Willen was that he had successfully treated patients with autoimmune diseases for at least a decade. We gave Courtney the allergy blood test he recommended, and, sure enough, she was eating many foods she was allergic to. We changed her diet and took her off all wheat and oat products. For a few months, we also took her off all milk products.

Dr. Willen gave me a book on leaky gut syndrome, explaining that the allergy-causing foods she was eating were probably irritating her immune system, which made her body attack her liver. He also sent me home with a regimen of his own supplements that included some of the amino acids and ALA that I was already giving her. He added a strong probiotic that was not milk based. He also agreed with Dr. Jordan Rubin about the efficacy of his Garden of Life supplements.

Suddenly it all seemed to come together! And it sounded logical. With all the doctors that I found, the common denominator seemed to be a glutathione-raising protocol and a massive improvement in Courtney's diet.

We completely changed from the standard American diet to one containing organic whole foods that were alkaline. And *absolutely no processed foods*. (Do you know how hard it is for a junior high school student not to eat fast food?) But Courtney needed to strengthen her immune system by raising the glutathione in every cell in her body. So that meant eliminating allergenic foods and eating more nutritious meals.

I already knew Courtney was allergic to milk because when she was younger she vomited it up, but her body was able to tolerate small amounts of cheese and ice cream. I had also read in Dr. Jordan Rubin's books that wheat was a major contributor to the poor nutrition and allergies in America, not just in the Otten household.

All of my researching and interrogating doctors was coming to a head. Dr. Willen solidified my conviction that there was a natural treatment for AIH. I just had to put all the pieces together, make the dietary changes, and give Courtney better supplements than the ones she'd been taking. Clearly, she hadn't been getting proper nutrition for the past twelve years. (I'm embarrassed to admit that I actually thought that feeding her "gummy bear" vitamins and "gumball vitamins" was going to help her stay healthy.)

It seemed that the doctors I had recently found all believed that if Courtney strengthened her compromised immune system with nutrients her body was lacking, then her body would function optimally and she'd regain her health. Hallelujah! Questions I had been asking Dr. Z. for five years were finally being answered by four independent doctors.

The alpha lipoic acid, the glyconutrient powder, and the other nineteen vitamins we gave Courtney were supposed to strengthen her immune system. Once they kicked in, we were confident that her body should be able to heal itself without the immune-suppressant drugs. The two doctors who had the greatest impact on my decisions were Dr. Berkson, whose practice in New Mexico helps patients by combining intravenous treatments of ALA and other nutraceuticals and nutrients, and Dr. Douglas Willen, whose wellness center in midtown Manhattan also advocates ALA and several other supplements plus strict dietary changes that emphasize avoiding allergenic foods. Dr. Berkson's research in conjunction with the National Institute of Health (NIH) postulates that ALA raises glutathione levels and regenerates the liver. Jo Bean from Oklahoma is still alive because of Dr. Berkson, and Kortni Gerhi was on the mend back in 2007 and 2008.

Next, I decided to add Dr. Willen's protocol to Courtney's regimen, so now we were combining Dr. Berkson's amazing ALA and supplements with the glyconutrients that Drs. Mondoa and McDonald endorsed, along with the nutrients that Dr. Willen suggested. In addition, Courtney was not going to eat wheat or dairy or any other foods that her blood work indicated were not good for her system.

In order to accomplish all this, I e-mailed Jo Bean in Oklahoma and Kortni in California and asked them what supplements that Dr. Berkson had sent them home with, along with the dosages and where to purchase them. I've learned that it's imperative to use high-quality supplements and nutraceuticals, as opposed to cheap ones you can pick up at the local grocery store.

Next, I had to figure out the proper dosage to give Courtney, who was still a young girl, so she couldn't take an adult dosage. When I compared the lists of supplements from my two new friends, I adjusted their dosages to suit Courtney's weight, as they were both heavier and older than my twelve-year-old. In August, 2007, I added Dr. Willen's protocol to her regimen. By this time, I was giving Courtney twenty-one supplements and nutraceuticals a day and taking her for lab work every two weeks. Now it was a test of time. I estimated that if I didn't find an answer for Courtney within three months (starting June 29, 2007), her liver could likely get worse and she would have to go on the leukemia meds or worse, the liver transplant list.

Most of my friends and clients who believe in Western medicine, thought I was nuts. But I didn't listen to those naysayers. This was my daughter who could die young, not theirs. Besides, I was following what Courtney's blood work was telling me and sticking to a protocol that already saved the lives of people who were treated by Dr. Berkson and Dr. Willen.

When I was searching the Internet for information on Dr. Burt Berkson in 2007, I found his scientific reports on successfully treating liver disease and hepatitis C on www.pubmed.gov. I typed "Burton Berkson" in the search box and found several research reports that validate that ALA and LDN have been successful in reversing diabetes and cirrhosis of the liver, as well as bringing thyroid and pancreatic cancer into remission. A couple of years later, however, the reports on hepatitis C and other liver diseases were removed from that website, and I haven't been able to find them. While I'm thrilled that I can still read some of Berkson's reports, I wonder...who is editing the scientific studies for the public to read? The next parent who is researching answers for AIH and ALA won't be able to find all of them on this site anymore. Is it the American Medical Association? If so, they apparently don't want people to find the helpful reports on ALA. And why did the editors of this prestigious medical website delete some of Dr. Berkson's work if it was proving efficacious in reversing cirrhosis from liver disease? Many of the reports are missing.

You can draw your own conclusions.

CHAPTER 15

The Power of Belief in Healing

One thing I had to do was persuade Courtney to believe this new protocol could work. If I didn't have her emotional and mental cooperation, the antioxidant therapy might not be successful. I've always been a strong believer in the power of manifestation, even before I read *The Secret*. Many books validate that faith and belief are paramount in creating a healthy and prosperous life.

On June 29, 2007, therefore, I called Courtney into the kitchen and told her that Daddy and I had decided not to give her the doctor's new drugs because I believed I had found a woman who was healed of the exact same thing she had. I told Courtney, "I truly believe these nutraceuticals will heal you, but YOU must believe they will work or they won't work. Will you believe?"

She responded with an obligatory, "Yes, Mommy."

My voice now took on a more serious tone. "I'm not kidding," I said. "If you believe these supplements will heal you, I will give you *anything* you want for your birthday," which was coming up in August. "Absolutely anything! BUT you must believe they will work! I need your help here."

Her beautiful blue eyes widened with excitement. "Anything?"

"Yes, anything. But you must believe. That's the deal."

"Okay!" she squealed.

"So what do you want for your birthday?"

"I know what I want."

"What?" I was preparing myself for something expensive.

"I want those second row Yankee seats that you can get from your friend Doug," she said. "And I want a ball autographed by Derek Jeter," she added with an even bigger grin.

"Okay," I said, "I think I can get the second row Yankee tickets, but how about if Derek Jeter just waves at you?"

"Nope. I want a ball autographed by Derek Jeter."

Now I was thinking, Oh, boy, this is going to set me back financially. We're already spending about $600 to $1,000 a month on supplements and doctor's visits. How much am I going to have to spend on an original Derek Jeter baseball from a dealer? Well, this was what she wanted, so this was what I was going to get for her. Somehow.

"Okay," I said aloud. "It's a deal. But you have to *believe* that these supplements will work!"

"I will, Mommy. I promise." And she proceeded to take her two handfuls of supplements and her nutrient powder.

Every day, Courtney took her ALA and her twenty other vitamins. Every two weeks, we took a blood test that Dr. Z would read to determine if her liver levels were getting better or worse.

After two weeks on the first batch of pills and powder I'd received from Ladonna, Courtney's liver levels stopped rising. They were even a tad lower. Her AST/ALT liver levels went from 65/77 to 43/59. That was slightly miraculous. Of course, I was looking for anything positive and couldn't be sure it was working yet because she was still on 10 mg. of prednisone. So I went on with my search for the complete nutritional answer to AIH. Every day, at work and at home, I Googled and learned more about glutathione and people whose autoimmune diseases were reversed and in remission because they were able to raise this protein in their cells.

After the first two weeks, I was still not satisfied at the results of Courtney's blood tests, and of course Dr. Z. was telling me that it was normal for her liver levels to bounce around. He was not encouraging. He was also hinting that she would get worse if she wasn't on the Cellcept. I thanked him for his opinion, but I felt driven to follow the antioxidant protocol for at least three months. It seemed to me that Dr. Z. was nervous, that maybe he was afraid Courtney's health would decline and he would be responsible. After all, she was taking a bunch of vitamins and nutraceuticals that her mother found from some doctors he'd never heard of and based on a science he'd never bothered to learn about. I understood his concern. He was probably afraid of a lawsuit.

But I was determined to find a natural remedy and, by God, I had just found two people whose liver had been regenerated and immune system restored by something other than dangerous drugs. I wasn't going to let any man stand in the way of my daughter's progress, even if he was a specialist at one of the best children's hospitals in the United States.

It may sound like I'm a stubborn, crazy female, but my reasoning was that Dr. Z. was only trained in Western allopathic medicine and had no knowledge about the benefits of supplements and nutraceutical therapy or any other alternative medicine. I was going to follow my instincts for at least three months, and I told Dr. Z. this, but at the same time, I needed his help and cooperation with ordering and reading her blood work, as that was his expertise. So I told him that I would send him an official e-mail stating that he was "no longer responsible for my daughter's health as I had chosen a different route. But I would humbly appreciate if he would order and diagnose her blood tests for me for the next few months." He thanked me for that e-mail, which I sent as promised, and we kept the lines of communications open.

All the while, I was praying every day to God (some call it a higher power) to help Courtney's body respond quickly to the new protocol. I believed that this nutritional concoction would work. Now it was a waiting game. Will this regimen be successful?

CHAPTER 16

Yankee Magic in the House That Babe Built

August 14, 2007, was the Best Birthday Celebration Ever for Courtney. For her twelfth birthday, I was able to pull a favor from a dear friend on Wall Street, Doug Teitelbaum, who gave me free tickets to his second-row box seats, right behind the Yankee dugout at Yankee Stadium. While we hadn't kept in touch very much, Doug is one of those friends who can't say no to helping a kid. I called him in July and told him about Courtney's AIH and my promise to her, and he was quick to say, "Sure. Tell me when her birthday is, and I'll get you the tickets."

When he put me on hold, I started crying because of his generosity. Doug is one of those old friends who doesn't have time for small talk anymore because of his meteoric success in business, but I know that he has a big heart. I received the tickets in the mail the next day for a game that was near her birthday. I'm sure that to this day, he has no idea how much he contributed to Courtney's recovery. I'll be eternally grateful for his kindness.

One promise down, one big promise to go.

Although I knew I was probably going to find a Derek Jeter autographed ball somewhere on-line for hundreds of dollars, I had another idea. Since I was desperate to fulfill my daughter's dream and keep my promise, I tried to call a childhood friend from Queens, Raymond Negron, who worked for Reggie Jackson and the Yankees back in the 1970s. He was now a consultant for the Bronx Bombers and author of "Yankee Miracles, Life With The Boss and The Bronx Bombers."

Ray had been a family friend of ours for years, and I knew my sister Jackie and our cousin Penelope were still in touch with him from time to time. When we were teenagers, he could always get us free Yankee tickets if no one else was using them. I hadn't seen him for twenty-six years, but I was desperate to find someone who might be remotely close to Derek Jeter. Ray was always on the road with the Yankees, however, so he didn't have an office phone where I could reach him.

Since I was so preoccupied with taking care of Courtney and her brother and sister, plus working full-time, I finally stopped trying to contact Ray by phone. I figured he would be at the Yankee game in August. The big day finally arrived. Yankee

Stadium. Second-row seats near first base. Right over the dugout. Courtney brought her girlfriend Gionna to the game to celebrate her birthday with her dad and me. We arrived early so the girls could get autographs from the players. Courtney and Gionna were so excited to see the players up close that they immediately ran to the corner of the dugout where Andy Petit and Joba Chamberlain were signing autographs for a bunch of kids. We'd bought each of the girls a new baseball and a cap so they could stretch their arms out over the dugout and hopefully be picked by the players to get their ball autographed. Courtney and Gionna came back, giggling and elated over their pictures and baseballs signed by the Yankee players.

"Courtney," I said, "look at this! You've got two autographed Yankee balls. I've never gotten an autographed ball in my life. You are so lucky!"

"Yeah," she replied, "but they're not Derek Jeter balls."

"Give me a break, kid! Second row seats. Two autographed balls, I've never in my life had a day like this."

"But it's not Derek Jeter."

And at that moment, I realized that it was going to be a challenge to make her wish come true. I stood up and looked around to see if somehow I could find my childhood friend, Raymond Negron, on the field. Just before the game started, I finally spotted him in the middle of a crowd of photographers and sportscasters. He was standing at the end of the dugout near home plate. He looked the same, only without the 1970's mustache I remembered, plus shorter hair, and he was wearing a suit and tie.

"RAAAAAAYYYYYYY!" I screamed in my loudest New York voice. At this point in my life I was so desperate to keep my promise to Courtney that good manners and proper etiquette went right out the window.

After yelling his name, I stared at him until I caught his eye. Since he had no clue who I was, I flashed a flirtatious grin and waved him over toward me. How could he resist a pretty woman with an engaging smile? I suppose he thought I was an old girlfriend, since the smile on my face was about as big as it could be. When he was about six feet away on the field side of the dugout, I yelled, "Ray! It's me, Denise Gabay. Jackie's sister and Penelope's cousin!"

He was obviously thrilled to see an old friend, and with a welcoming grin said, "Hey, how are you, great to see you, and how's the family?"

I knew I had just about sixty seconds to tell him what I needed, so I gave him the condensed version of Courtney's story and said I was trying make her birthday wish come true with an autographed ball.

All he said was, "No problem, sweetie, I'll get you a ball from one of the Yankees and I'll come find you at the end of the game. Gotta go now, we'll talk later." And with that, he vanished into the dugout and the game began.

My heart was filled with joy. I had a great feeling that Ray was going to come through for me. Even though we hadn't seen each other in almost thirty years, I just felt it in my heart. Back in the old neighborhood, he had always been a generous kid and always kept his word whenever we asked him for Yankee tickets or a ride in his car.

But suddenly it hit me—I hadn't asked specifically for a Derek Jeter autographed ball. I stood there and squeezed my eyes shut and prayed as hard as I could that he'd bring us back a present from the Yankee captain.

The magic continued for Courtney. Between innings, when the sides retired and the Yankees came back into their dugout, Alex Rodriguez spotted Courtney's little blonde girlfriend, Gionna, and signaled to my husband to give her the ball he was about to throw to him. Mike nodded, A-Rod threw the ball, and Mike gave it to Gionna. Courtney and her buddy were screaming with glee. And of course, Gionna, being the great friend that she is, just turned to Courtney and gave her the ball.

"It's your birthday," she said. "You can have it.

I already have two signed balls and an autographed baseball cap."

"Look at that," I screamed to Courtney. "Now you've even got an Alex Rodriguez ball!"

She looked at me with her big, beautiful, blue eyes. "Yes. But it's not Derek Jeter."

"C'mon, kid," I shot back. "You're killing me! You've gotten everything I promised. And more!"

She smiled sweetly with those prednisone puffy cheeks, shook her head, and said, "Nope. I still want a Derek Jeter ball. That's what you promised."

I still had hopes that Ray would come through for me.

At the top of the ninth inning, the Yankees were losing miserably. Mike wanted to leave, but I said, "I'm not going until after the game is over and Ray comes to find us."

He asked if I thought he would really come, and I shot back, "Of course he will!"

I had faith in Ray. I remember my sister telling me that Ray had four kids of his own. How could he possibly deny my little pumpkin an autographed ball when she had that deadly disease?.

Then it was the bottom of the ninth. I kept looking for him on the field. Then I heard someone behind me call my name. I turned around, and there he was, tall, dark, and handsome as always, with his electrifying smile. He was holding a Yankee ball in his hand. My heart jumped. Could it be a Derek Jeter ball?

Ray made his way over to us, and I introduced him to Mike, Courtney, and Gionna. After our brief hugs and kisses and a quick update on the past twenty-six years, he turned to Courtney and handed her an autographed ball. Hideki Matsui.

She thanked him politely and turned to me and mouthed the words, *It's not Derek Jeter.*

At just that moment, Ray tapped her on the shoulder. As she turned again, he said, "Courtney, I'm sorry I couldn't get a ball for your girlfriend, I just didn't have time, and the Yankees are busy with the game. So I tell you what—I'll send you two balls in the mail next week signed by Derek Jeter."

I almost swallowed my tongue. Courtney and I looked at each other. What had we just heard? Her big blue eyes opened wider than I'd ever seen before and her jaw dropped open. I had tears in my eyes. We said a big thank you to Raymond, and Courtney hugged him tight. Raymond Negron never had any idea that Courtney had been hoping to get a Derek Jeter ball. He made her wish come true! He gave us a Magical Yankee Day.

After Ray left, Courtney turned to me. "I can't believe it!" she squealed, but I just pointed my finger at her.

"I kept my end of the bargain. You've gotten

everything you wanted for your birthday, now you HAVE to keep your end of the deal. YOU MUST GET BETTER. You promised!"

She couldn't contain her happiness. "Yes, mommy," she shrieked, "I promise, *I promise.*"

Her little round face was filled with such joy that at that moment I realized I was witnessing a true miracle. Everything my little girl had wished for was coming true. As my family and Gionna turned their attention back to the end of the game, I turned my head away and sat quietly and cried with joy. Then I looked up into the sky and quietly said, "Thank you, God. Thank you. What an amazing miracle!"

I'm not a religious person by traditional standards, but I have always had a strong belief in a higher power. Courtney's illness was my own personal foxhole in this war on autoimmune disease. I was reaching out to God and hoping for miracles and support to help me battle this AIH monster in a non-traditional way. That day in Yankee stadium, it was like God, (or the higher power by any other name) was telling me that everything was going to be OK.

Two weeks later, Courtney received a box in the mail from Raymond Negron. As she ripped open the box, her smile was as big as it was that day in Yankee Stadium. In the box were the two promised Derek Jeter autographed balls. We looked at each other in disbelief again, just like we had at the game, only now we were both smiling so hard our cheeks were hurting.

"I kept my promise," I said again, "and you've gotten everything you asked for. Now you have to keep your promise and get better."

She looked at me. Her grin couldn't have been any larger. "I promise, Mommy, I promise."

I felt like I was in the 1992 movie, *The Babe,* where we see Babe Ruth with the dying kid, Johnny, who asks him to hit a home run in the 1926 World Series and raise his spirits. But this was real life. It was surreal life. Courtney ran into her room with her prized baseballs to check on the Internet to see if the autograph was an authentic Derek Jeter signature.

I stood alone in the kitchen. Again, I looked up toward God and whispered, "Thank you, God, oh my God, thank you."

The miracles kept happening.

That was the end of August, 2007, and she was still on 10 mgs. of prednisone and twenty-one different supplements every day. September came, the kids went back to school, and everything stayed the same. Her blood tests still showed little improvement and her AST/ALT levels remained at 70/80. This was still too high for the body of an 85-pound child. All of a sudden, it didn't seem like the Yankee miracle was working. I got depressed again.

Then in mid-September, the Jewish high holy days rolled around. These holy days, Yom Kippur and Rosh Hashana, are as important as Easter and Ramadan are for Christians and Muslims. But suddenly I was not in a mood to honor God, as I felt he had abandoned me and (for whatever reason) wasn't allowing my baby girl to get better. Frankly, I felt that if God was going to let my daughter die at an early age, I couldn't honor him on any holiday. As far as the doctors were concerned, Courtney should now be on Cellcept, a strong leukemia drug, before she got worse. The thought of my twelve-year-old daughter having a liver transplant in the near future was too much to bear.

I was angry with God. A few days before Rosh Hashana, I found myself alone in my kitchen, trying to decide if I wanted to celebrate the high holy holidays. I looked up at the ceiling, as if I could see God up above, and with tears streaming down my face I screamed at him.

"I'm not going to celebrate any holy days until you show me a miracle! I know you can perform miracles. Now help my daughter get better." I was shaking my fist at the invisible God. I shouted louder than before, "I know you can do it! Please make Courtney better. I can't take it anymore, I just can't handle it anymore!"

And then, I calmed down and decided I was going to boycott God and all Jewish holidays until my daughter was better.

Now if you're a practicing Jew, Christian, Muslim, or a member of any other religion, you know that not honoring God on a high holy day might be considered blasphemous...or worse. But I was exhausted. I had been praying and begging and crying every night for months. Now, I said to myself, I'd had my last conversation with God until my daughter got better. I felt abandoned by the Almighty. I had the love and strength of my husband and my parents and family, of course, but I was worn out. I was running out of options. I knew—intellectually—that there was a small chance of her recovering because my friend Ladonna Jones recovered completely, and she had been on the liver transplant list. But my faith was waning. I couldn't pray anymore. My energy was depleted. Celebrating was the last thing I wanted to do. God was taking my daughter away from me, and I hated it. There was no way I was honoring him this year. I was done with God.

Life continued as it always did in the Otten household. All three children were back in school and busy with homework, sports, and dance lessons, and I also had my full-time job as a financial advisor in a Wall Street firm. These weren't good times, but I was still pushing forward and looking for validation that these supplements would help my beautiful little girl, who was still puffy from the prednisone.

On September 27, 2007, Courtney and I made our

regular visit to the local lab to get her blood tested. Back in July, her liver levels had shown a slight improvement, with her AST/ALT levels at a low of 43/59. But the doctors were not impressed because at the very next blood test her levels shot up to 63/79. Then they went up to 74/88. I didn't care what Dr. Z. said, I wasn't ready to give up hope. Normal AST/ALT liver levels are around the low 20s, but Courtney's hovered between 50 and 90 while she was still taking 10 mgs. of prednisone. At least they hadn't gone into the 100 level for the past two and a half months. As always, I dropped Courtney off at school after her test. The next day I got my customary phone call from the nurse at Dr. Z.'s office.

"Hi, Mrs. Otten. It's Nurse Y, calling about Courtney's lab work."

My heart sank and my throat choked up as I slid off my chair and dropped to my knees beside my desk in one more attempt to beg God for a miracle.

"I have great news for you!" said the nurse. I held my breath and closed my eyes. "Courtney's blood test came back," she said. "And it's great, really great. Her AST/ALT levels are down to normal—23/25. They're the best they've been in five years!"

I couldn't help it. I started crying. Right there, on my knees in my office, I started crying. "Are you sure?" I asked her. "Can you repeat that? I want to write down the numbers to tell my husband."

She repeated the numbers, then added, "Yes, the blood work is perfect. She's doing great."

All I could say was, "Thank you, thank you. And," I quickly added, "please thank the doctor for helping me with the blood work for all these months." I couldn't say thank you enough. I just kept saying it over and over again.

Finally I hung up, got up off the floor, and immediately called Mike. "Are you sitting down?" I asked him.

"Yes."

"I just got a call from the nurse at the hospital. She said Courtney's liver levels are normal. They're 23/25!"

Mike was so happy to hear this, I could practically see the big smile on his face through the phone. He laughed out loud. "That's incredible. Oh my god, that's great news! I can't believe it. All that research and all those vitamins and nutraceuticals actually worked. Maybe we should be taking them." He stopped a minute, then added, " Hon, you missed your calling. You should have been a doctor."

I lovingly thanked him for the recognition, and then thought to myself, I think it was my training as a financial advisor that served me well to research and uncover a scientifically valid alternative protocol for this deadly disease.

Neither of us wanted to wait to tell Courtney, but

we had to wait until after school. Before we hung up, Mike and I both said, "I love you." But this time it was more than that simple declaration you give your spouse before getting off the phone. There was a big non-verbal hug attached this time because together, as a family, we were beating that god-awful disease that could have taken our daughter from us.

After I hung up with Mike, my body felt limp. I slumped in my chair. Then I looked up at the ceiling. "Thank you, God!" I called out. "Thank you. I'm sorry I didn't believe in you."

Then I called my mom, my dad and my step mom, and mother-in-law to tell them about Courtney's levels. I'm not sure they understood how amazing this news was, however, because I had never told them that Courtney could die from AIH. I had never wanted to utter the words *she could die* out loud to anyone. At the time, I also didn't have the energy to finally explain the seriousness of the situation. I still had to call the rest of my family and all of our friends who knew about the severity of Courtney's illness.

My mom, who has always lovingly supported my research and holistic way of life, just kept repeating, "Oh my God, congratulations, darling. Thank God, thank God."

My dad and his wife, Fran, who are like most people and believe in traditional medical therapy, were also happy for us and thrilled that we had finally found an answer for Courtney's illness. They are the type of parents who will support you emotionally, 150 percent, in anything you choose. But to heal a body without traditional medicine and not listen to the best doctors in America was incomprehensible to them. I think they were more surprised than anyone else in my family that the alternative therapy had worked. .

Then there's my mother-in-law, Beverly, a devout Christian who has been a vitamin advocate for decades, but like everyone in America would never go against the doctor's orders. What did she say? She confidently told me, "I knew God would take care of her, and I just had faith that you were going to do the right thing."

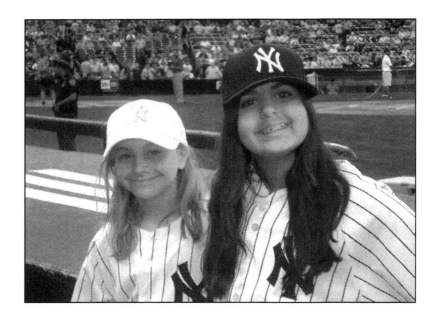

Courtney partially puffy, at Yankee Stadium

CHAPTER 17

Breaking the News To My Little Girl

Finally it was time to break the news to our "Cordy-Bear." At 2:45, as soon as I thought she would be home from school, I phoned Courtney on her cell phone and told her that the blood work came back normal. As you might imagine, being a typical twelve-year-old who was absorbed in her schoolwork and social life, she didn't seem particularly surprised.

In fact, she responded to my earth-shaking news like it was no big deal, which I thought was pretty amusing, as I had been crying and praying and doing research every day since the doctor told us the Imuran and the standard treatment failed. Not to mention living in fear for four and a half years that my youngest child might die.

At the same time, I wasn't shocked at her reaction as I had never told her the whole truth about her health. I'd always told her as much as she needed to know at the time.

What I never told Courtney was that AIH was

a life-threatening disease for sixty percent of the people who get it (according to the statistics in 2007). I had never told her she could die from it. I've been reading self-help books for over twenty years, books by authors who teach the principles of the power of the mind, like Louise Hay, Dr. Bernie Siegel, Deepak Chopra, Dr. Wayne Dyer, and (more recently) Gregg Braden and Dr. Bruce Lipton. These authors recommend that you *not* tell the sick person that they could die from the disease. You should always help them believe that they will get better. You should help them see themselves as well. Belief is a tremendous part of the healing process. Also of great importance is that you should constantly give the patient lots of love, repeat uplifting positive affirmations, and indulge in laughter and good nutrition. All of this advice is essential to maintaining a healthy body. It also seems easier to convince a child that she is already well. Adults have so much emotional baggage that it's more difficult to persuade a fifty-year-old that their doctor might be wrong and they can help themselves if they change their thought patterns and beliefs. It's often not too hard to convince a child who's loved and generally happy that she will get better if she just believes she's getting well. Most kids just want to have fun, fun, fun. And that's my Courtney. She's always been a happy soul.

There are many people who have autoimmune diseases, specifically autoimmune hepatitis or hepatitis C, and all the cancers that Dr. Berkson has success with, who could benefit from this antioxidant protocol. I'm not professing to have "the answer" to help every person with AIH, however, nor do I believe I have the panacea to reverse the symptoms of all autoimmune diseases. Everyone can decide what kind of treatment is best for them. It's a personal choice. But I do believe that the supplement and nutraceutical therapy that I learned from four doctors—Berkson, Willen, Mondoa, and McDonald—is what healed my daughter. The alternative therapy is the reason that, as I write this, my Courtney is healthy, tall, gorgeous and brilliant.

Well, of course, getting her birthday wishes also made her happy. For this little girl, Derek Jeter and Yankee baseball were her major passion. Whatever your passion is, go for it. Learn to be as happy as a kid again. We should all take a lesson from this and try to live life every day with love and exuberance.

Having said that, I know that everyone is different. Our friend Ladonna Jones was in complete remission from AIH within nine months after she began a similar alternative protocol. My friend Jo Bean's Hep C is in remission because of Dr. Berkson's antioxidant therapy and an inexpensive drug called low-dose naltrexone. Our other friend, the beautiful blonde Kortni Gehri, who has AIH, had to have a liver transplant at age twenty-five. Her liver transplant saved her life, and as I write this, she is studying to be a nurse.

While everyone and every body heals differently, I believe it's critical to know about your choices. Just believing what the Federal Drug Administration says is the only way to reverse your illness may not serve you and your body. But following the FDA's advice may create millions of dollars for the FDA and the pharmaceutical industry. (And who among us can believe what federal government agencies say is true these days?)

My advice? Choose your medical practitioners wisely. Do your homework. Use the Internet to find books written or endorsed by doctors who have had great success in the area you're interested in. Go to www.pubmed.gov and other internet sites to cross reference your research. If you're too frozen with fear because of your diagnosis to even think about an alternative remedy, ask a friend or family member to go on the Internet and do some research for you. And don't hesitate to call a doctor's office to find out if they've had success with your particular disease. Then press them to explain their alternative protocol.

Also, after you talk to your doctor, don't hesitate to get a second opinion. Or a third opinion. You must find the doctor you agree with and who will treat you with kindness and respect. Don't worry about firing doctors who don't make you feel comfortable. You can exit their office gracefully as you say, "Thank you for all of your help."

One big lesson I learned from Courtney's healing came from a dear friend named Frank Valanzola. I met Frank when we were both financial advisors at that big Wall Street firm. He was one of the supportive friends I could call and cry to when Courtney was ill and my family was feeling overwhelmed. When I met Frank in 2005, he was a brain cancer survivor and had a strong will to live. He was one of the first ten people I called to share the good news of Courtney's healing.

"I knew you would do it!" he said. "I had faith in you."

And then, three years later, his cancer came back. It metastasized into his lungs, then all over his body. He was given a year to a year and a half to live. Frank believed in the traditional chemotherapy and radiation treatment and nothing else. That regimen had healed him in 2005, so he had no reason to believe it shouldn't help him again. And of course he went to a man who is arguably the best oncologist in New York.

Even though he saw me go through a devastating year with Courtney's health, and he and his wife joined our family celebration of Courtney's Bat Mitzvah in 2008 after her AIH was in remission because of this antioxidant protocol, Frank never wanted to call an alternative M.D. for a holistic consultation. He wouldn't even consider going a nutritional, non-traditional route. There was nothing I could do to convince him. Eventually I had to stop trying. This was his life, I reluctantly told myself, and his choice, and he was a proud man. He only believed in whatever the FDA recommended.

In September, 2011, Frank lost his battle to cancer. He was only fifty-one years old, six months older than me. As his friend, I was there to give emotional support to him and his wife Deborah, plus any laughter I could muster up for him. But I had to honor his decision to use the doctors he thought were right for him, no matter what...even though I vehemently disagreed. It was his life.

My lesson is a humble one. While I was able to find an answer for my daughter's AIH, and work with great doctors, too, I learned that we must allow others the freedom to make their own choices for their health. I could help Courtney because I'm her mother and can make decisions for her as long as she's a child. I was responsible for her health. But I couldn't help Frank. I still wonder what would have happened if he had sought out an alternative M.D.

who had success with his type of cancer. Now we will never know.

All we can do is offer the information and scientific evidence to our friends, family, and the public. Then we have to allow them to decide for themselves. So here, my friends, is the information. Please see the books listed at the end of this book. If you need more information, please go to my website, www. curingcourtney.com, to find more holistic modalities and doctors to interview. And then read, read, read!

CHAPTER 18

Courtney's Antioxidant Protocol and Diet

For those who have been waiting to find out exactly what I gave Courtney and to take a peek at her lab results, here they are. If you're ill, however, I must advise you to work with an M.D. who can follow your progress with a bi-monthly blood test and monitor your vitamin and nutraceutical intake. Or find a doctor who has had both long-term experience and success with alternative therapies. See if you can speak to any of their patients who have been healed. My darling Kortni Gehri tried several alternative therapies from medical practitioners that were said to have been successful for some patients, but were unsuccessful for her. Ultimately, the liver transplant was her only answer. So be smart and do your homework. My website has a list of reputable physicians and health practitioners who are familiar with alternative therapies. I welcome your thoughts and inquiries.

The following list gives the supplements and nutraceuticals that helped my daughter get well. She took half the daily dose in the morning and half at night.

- 600 mg. per day of alpha lipoic acid (ALA) The brand recommended by Dr. Burt Berkson back in 2007 was Biotech. He has done his research on the quality of the ALA.

- 100 mg. B-complex. (Take this because ALA absorbs vitamin B.) Twice a day.

- Fungal/Primal Defense (non-milk probiotic.) (A Garden of Life product from Dr. Jordan Rubin.) Two pills a day.

- High quality children's multi vitamins. (No grocery store vitamins!) Two a day.

- Silymarin (also known as milk thistle) Biotech brand. (Note that some Silymarin can be detrimental to the system if the capsules are filled with talc. Be sure to get a good quality milk thistle) one daily.

- Selenium, 100 mcg (Biotech). Two a day.

- Omega 3-6-9, Nordic Natural Fish Oil (1000 mg.) Two a day.

- A/O (anti-oxidant) amino acids. (Mannitech brand.) Two pills a day.

- Classic Ambrotose (Mannitech.) Two tablespoons a day (in juice.)

I adjusted Courtney's diet by eliminating what she was very allergic to and introduced her to only whole organic foods. If I gave her pasta (which is a processed food), I used only non-wheat/gluten-free pasta.

Here is a sample of the diet Dr. Berkson recommended to his patient Joanna Bean. I already had my other daughter on a similar regimen, minus the allergy-producing foods, so when Jo sent me this list, I just smiled and realized that I had just strayed off the nutritional path a bit too much when Courtney was born. This diet wasn't foreign to me, I just had to follow it more carefully.

- *Six green vegetables a day, ½ cup serving. Includes asparagus, kohlrabi, artichoke, summer squash, leeks, snow peas, green beans, wax beans, bean sprouts, beets, mushrooms, broccoli, brussels sprouts, cabbage, cauliflower, okra, onions, eggplant, kale, greens, parsnips, tomatoes, turnips, peapods, cucumber, celery, peppers, radishes, sweet potatoes, romaine lettuce (no iceberg!), hot peppers (chilis), rutabaga, carrots, beets (sparingly due to iron).*

- *Whole grains, ½ cup serving. Includes oatmeal, brown rice, buckwheat, rye bread, grits, corn, whole grains. I added to this list:*

millet, quinoa, amaranth. No boxed cereals! (Courtney eliminated wheat)

• *Proteins, serving size = the palm of your hand. Includes chicken, turkey (roasted), fish (grilled or baked), beans (not canned), lamb, seafood, eggs, wild game, Non-processed cheese, tofu.*

• *Oils and fats. Includes olive oil, coconut oil, butter, fish oil, black currant oil, flax seed oil.*

• *Fruits, serving size, ½ cup. Includes apples, natural applesauce, apricots, bananas, berries (strawberries, blueberries, raspberries blackberries, cherries, grapes, kiwi, nectarines, oranges, papaya, mango, plum, pear, peach, pineapple, tangerine, pomegranate.*

• *Fluids. 6-8 glasses of water a day, coffee (no more than 2 cups a day), tea, herb tea, seltzer water with a little juice, no more than 1-2 glasses of no-sugar-added fruit juice a day.*

• *Raw sugar and honey in moderation*

Avoid the Following:

- Milk by the glass, no low-fat or skim milk

- White flour, sugar

- Tobacco, alcohol

- Salty foods

- Soft drinks especially diet sodas

- Margarine and most cooking oils

- Processed foods, deep fried foods

- Grapefruit

- Peanuts in any form

- Tylenol/acetaminophen

Must Do:

- Exercise

- Stress reduction program

- Bowel movement every day

- Get 15 minutes of sunshine daily

- HAVE FUN. Keep a positive attitude

Although every patient's ailment and diet are different, this was—and still is—a good diet (minus the wheat and milk) for Courtney and her friend Gionna, who has celiac disease. Nutraceuticals and supplements also vary from patient to patient.

There are dozens of whole food diets popular in the nutritional community. This is only one healthy way of eating. Again, I eliminated the foods Courtney is allergic to. However, if you read the books by Dr. Jordan Rubin you will find that his dietary restrictions are a bit different. The diet recommended by Dr. Douglas Willen is the Paleo diet which doesn't have grains in it at all and includes lots of meat. Then there is the popular book The China Study, by Dr. T. Colin Campbell who expounds on the benefits produced by a plant-based diet. He believes that all sorts of chronic diseases like heart disease, cancer, diabetes, stroke, hypertension, arthritis, alzheimer's, and others can largely be prevented by change in diet based on his long-term research. The common thread in most nutritional diets is that they honor whole foods and follow an organic protocol. You should find the diet that suits your allergies and work with a health care practitioner who's had great success with your illness. Remember, every body type and blood type is different. You must seek out what is right for your body. Your body is your temple, take care of it. None of this is approved by the FDA, of course, but the friends who helped me were all working with professionals who had been successful at treating their patients. Don't go out and start buying every supplement on this list and expect your disease to disappear. Find an expert in this field who can assist you. Or contact me via my website, and I'll help you find a doctor in your area.

On October 16, 2007, after a few weeks of perfect blood work, Courtney's labs showed her AST/ALT levels at 25/25. At that point I told Dr. Z. that I was going to wean her off the prednisone. That's when he suggested doing it their way, slowly and half a pill every two weeks. I cooperated with this weaning protocol, and on December 3, 2007, Dr. Z. took Courtney off all of the prednisone. Her AST/ALT liver levels continued to be in the mid- to high-20s the last three months: 28/22, 28/26, 23/22.

As you can see from the pictures in this book, Courtney has grown into a gorgeous young woman who is a great athlete, student, sister, and daughter. She is in great health and stronger than her mom.

Imagine if every doctor in the United States were taught about not only medicine, but also nutrition and the power of belief. It is shortsighted and scientifically illogical to believe that only one methodology can heal. We must explore all possibilities. In this world of new technologies and advanced scientific study, it's also illogical to believe that the American Medical Association has ALL the answers. They only have a few. There are dozens of methods of healing, and everyone's body responds differently to any method. It's up to each patient to do his or her due diligence if he or she expects to lead a healthy life.

My hope and prayer is that I can help other people find alternative answers for autoimmune diseases for their children and themselves. Don't just pop a pill and think that will reverse a severe disease. Find out how to get your body back to its original healthy state. What fundamental nutrients are you deficient in that created this dis-ease? Work with a medical professional and an alternative physician to find what works best for you. You may need medication to stop the bleeding while you simultaneously introduce the supplements and nutraceuticals to reverse your failing health so your body can get back to normal. Your objective is ALWAYS to improve your immune system. Don't just accept a traditional medical protocol because the doctor says so. Do your research! Ask yourself, why go under the knife until you've exhausted all your alternative options?

I'm eternally grateful to the inventors of Google, Yahoo, and other Internet search engines. I found my answer from the people, doctors, research data, and books I found online. Don't stop surfing the Net until you find the answers to your questions.

And by all means, trust your intuition and powers of intellectual deductive reasoning. Be your own warrior, whether it's for your health or that of your child's.

Three years after Courtney was in remission we finally admitted to her that Autoimmune Hepatitis was a life threatening illness and that she was somewhat in danger of having a liver transplant which could lead to an early death. Obviously she was shocked at the news and asked me "why didn't you tell me this before?" I replied emphatically, "if you tell a person they are going to die, they will likely believe you." "But," I added, "if I tell you that you'll get better soon, you'll probably believe it instead." She nodded in agreement and said, "yeah, you're right about that."

Recently Courtney shared with me HER interpretation of why she got better when the doctors couldn't help her. As a young girl she always believed she would get back to normal. One of the lessons she learned from this ordeal was that with determination and the support of family and friends one can conquer the unthinkable. Courtney truly believes that what a person is capable of lies in their will. And I've witnessed her iron will on the softball field when there's 2 outs and she's the batter up at the end of a game. Oftentime, she would get a base hit to keep the game alive and ignore the pressure from her coaches and teammates, validating her belief within that she would hit the ball no matter what. My interpretation is that the supplements helped her BUT it was Courtney who had the powerful desire to make it happen.

If you ask my three kids, you'll get a different opinion. Adam, Cara and Courtney all wrote essays in high school on their experience of Courtney's miraculous remission. Each of them (without the others knowing) described their mother as "she's nobody special, not famous or super rich, but she's amazing because she found the answer to help Courtney get better."

Out of the mouths of babes. They are telling you that if I can do it, so can you.

Autoimmune Hepatitis Flowsheet

Patient: Courtney Bitten

MRN 472-84-031

DOB -08/02/1993

Date	AST	ALT	GGT	AlkPhos	T/D bili	T.prot/Alb	Amy/Lip	Na	K	Cl	HCO3	BUN	Cr	Gluc	WBC	H/H	plt	T-4 prednisone	Drug Dose Imuran	Cellcept

Patient: Otten, Courtney

MRN: 472-84-03

Diagnosis

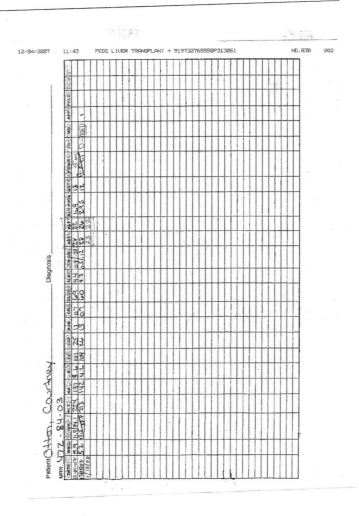

NYC hospital lab sheets

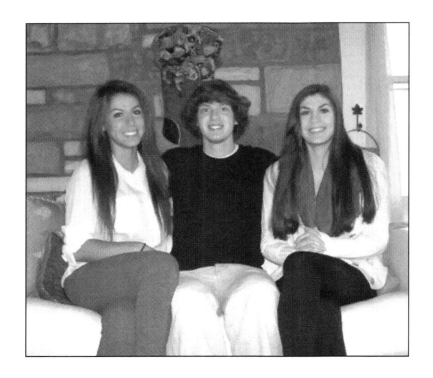

My kids

CHAPTER 19

So the Question Remains....

What reversed my Courtney's illness? Was it the multitude of supplements that I put together from the protocols of four different doctors? Or was it that Courtney's young, impressionable mind and heart genuinely believed that she was going to be well because she was ecstatically happy when she got her wish fulfilled with second row seats at Yankee Stadium and two autographed Derek Jeter baseballs? Was it at that time that the biology of belief changed her cellular structure so her autoimmune system started working within my arbitrary three-month timeframe?

Everyone has their opinion. The doctor at the famous children's hospital in New York City told me that "the meds kicked in," and that was the reason her liver levels went back to normal. I think not. Otherwise, why would he have prescribed the leukemia drug, Cellcept?

Was it the supplements and nutraceuticals or the

magic of Courtney's happiness at Yankee Stadium?
What do you believe?

I wish you love, light, health, and prosperity.

Love,
Courtney's mom, Denise

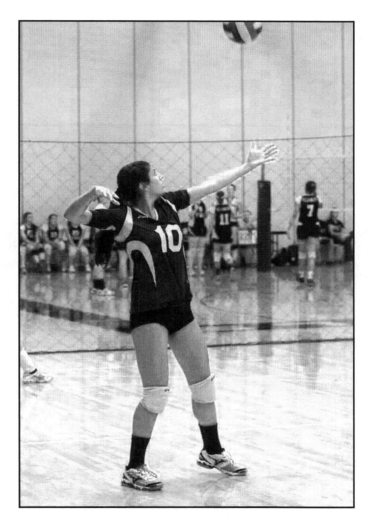

Courtney, slim and athletic, the antithesis of sickness

Photo courtesy of Alexandra Wildmoser-Todd

READING LIST

Berkson, M.D., Burt. *The Alpha Lipoic Breakthrough: The Superb Antioxidant That May Slow Aging, Repair Liver Damage, And Reduce The Risk of Cancer, Heart Disease And Diabetes*, Three Rivers Press, New York, New York, 1998

Braden, Gregg. *The Devine Matrix: Bridging Time, Space, Miracles And Belief*. Hay House, Inc., 2007.

Campbell, Ph.D., T. Colin and Thomas M. Campbell II. *The China Study: Startling Implications for Diet, Weight Loss and Long-Term Health*. Benbella Books, Inc., Dallas, Texas, 2006.

D'Adamo, M.D., Peter J., and Catherine Whitney. *Eat Right 4 Your Type: The Individualized Diet Solution. G.P. Putnam's & Sons, New York, N.Y., 2006.*

Habakus, MA, Louise Kuo. and Mary Holland. *Vaccine Epidemic: How Corporate Greed, Biased Science, and Coercive Government Threaten Our Human rights, Our Health, and Our Children.* Skyhorse Publishing, New York, N.Y., 2011

Hay, Louise. *You Can Heal Your Life,* by Hay House, Inc., 1999

Kaufmann, Doug A., and Beverly Thornhill Hunt, Ph.D. *The Fungus Link: An Introduction to Fungal Disease Including The Initial Phase Diet.* Rockwall, Texas: MediaTrition, 2000.

Lipton, PhD., Bruce H. *The Biology of Belief: Unleashing The Power of Conciousness, Matter & Miracles.* Hay House, Inc., 2008.

Mondoa, M.D., Emil. *Sugars That Heal: The New Healing Science of Glyconutrients*, Published by Random House Publishing Group, 2001.

McCarthy, Jenny. *Louder Than Words: A Mother's Journey In Healing Autism.* Dutton, A Member of Penguin Group (USA), Inc., 2007.

Rubin, Jordan S. *The Maker's Diet: The 40-Day Health Experience That Will Change Your Life Forever.* Siloam, a Strang Company, Lake Mary, Florida, 2004, 2005.

Siegel, M.D., Bernie S. *Love, Medicine & Miracles: Lessons Learned about Self-Healing from a Surgeon's Experience with Exceptional Patients.* Harper & Row Publishers, Inc., N.Y.C, N.Y., 1986.

Schopick, Julia. *Honest Medicine: Effective, Time-Tested, Inexpensive Treatments for Life Threatening Diseases.* Published by Innovative Health Publishing, Oak Park, Illinois., 2011.

Resource List

NEW JERSEY

David Barrett, III, D.C.,
Denville Chiropractic/Sports & Rehab
161 East Main Street
Denville, NJ 07834
(973) 627-0910

Gary Klingsberg, D.O.
Center for Nutrition and Preventive Medicine
177 North Dean Street
Englewood, NJ 07631
(201) 503-0007

Paula Gotthelf, Nutritionist
42 King Place
Closter, NJ 07624
(201) 280-2742

Mark Morris, D.O.
26 Milburn Ave.
Springfield, N.J.
973-258-1776

Elaine Hardy, MS, RN, APN
319 Airport Rd.
Hackettstown, N.J. 07840
(903) 850-0888

NEW MEXICO

Burton Berkson, M.D., Ph.D
Integrative Medical Center of N.M
1155 Commerce Dr. #C
Las Cruces, N.M. 88011
(575) 524-3720

NEW YORK

Ronald Hoffman, M.D.
The Hoffman Center
776 Sixth Avenue, Suite 4B
New York, NY 10001
(212) 779-1744

Douglas Willen, D.C.
Willen Wellness Center
900 Broadway #403
New York, NY 10003
(347) 371-2715

TEXAS

Ladonna Jones, Mannatech Sales Associate
http://mymannapages.com/esuite/home/cljones

ACKNOWLEDGEMENTS

I want to send unconditional thanks and love to many people who contributed not only to this book, but to helping me find the alternative anti-oxidant protocol that allowed Courtney to become the healthy and beautiful young woman that you see on this cover. Starting with Dr. Burt Berkson, Dr. Doug Willen, and adding to that my posse of ladies who I called constantly for their guidance and support: Ladonna Jones, Mary Jo Bean, Susie and Kortni Gehri. Without them, I don't think I would have a healthy Courtney today!

A big thanks to my book mentor Julia Schopick, author of *Honest Medicine*, who inspired me to push forward. The great editing by Barbara Ardinger, Ph.D, the publishing brilliance of Jose Ramirez and Barbara Rainess at Pedernales Publishing and my superb book cover Artist George Foster and his wife Mary of Foster Covers are people to be applauded. The tender love between a mother and daughter was captured by my outstanding photographer Anthony Grasso and make-up artist Terese Broccoli. Their artistic talents were able to reveal Courtney's natural beauty so that the readers can appreciate what a true miracle looks like when science and belief come together to reverse a deadly childhood disease.

The most grateful thank you goes to my friends and entire family for supporting my quirky efforts of wanting to find an alternative remedy for my daughter when we all suspected her future was bleak. My sisters Jackie and Michele, and Cousin Penelope were always there to lend an ear and never judged my request for more holistic information from them. The New Jersey mothers who helped make Courtney feel like nothing was wrong, gave her the love that she needed while I struggled to find an answer. My parents and mother-in-law, Evelyn, Henry, Francine, and Beverly were always in my corner because they respected my judgment and knew how much Courtney was loved and protected by her parents. But the biggest hugs go out to my little Otten household. My husband, who has had to deal with my "always being a little different than other wives," has been my rock when I crumble. We've cried together and cheered together when going through this ordeal. I couldn't have asked for a more loving husband and father of our kids. And, of course, my three blessed children. They stuck by their mother, even when they thought I was a little too crazy and excessive with nutrition. And when it looked like Courtney's life was hard because of the drug-induced body changes, Adam and Cara took care of her when Mom and Dad weren't there. Petite Cara got into some fights to defend her sister, and Adam protected her like a bodyguard. But the one person who deserves the deepest bow is my gorgeous blue-eyed Courtney. Without her unbelievable strength to survive and thrive this book would have blank pages. She is my hero. I always will admire her endless positive attitude. I hope Courtney's pre-teen struggle and this book will give others hope that some autoimmune diseases can have a happy ending.

Made in the USA
Lexington, KY
31 October 2019